THE SOCIAL RESPONSIBILITY
OF GYNECOLOGY AND OBSTETRICS

THE SOCIAL RESPONSIBILITY
of Gynecology and Obstetrics

Edited with Introductions by
ALLAN C. BARNES

{ PROCEEDINGS OF A CONFERENCE
HELD MAY 7, 1965, AT
THE JOHNS HOPKINS HOSPITAL }

The Johns Hopkins Press, Baltimore
1965

TO OUR GRANDCHILDREN
AND TO THEIR GRANDCHILDREN

FOR ONLY BY DEDICATING OUR
THOUGHTFUL EFFORTS ON THEIR BEHALF
CAN WE SUCCESSFULLY MOLD A SOCIETY FIT
TO RECEIVE THEM, OR INDEED CREATE
CITIZENS FIT TO BE BORN.

PARTICIPANTS

ALLAN C. BARNES, M.D.

Professor and Director of the Department of Gynecology and Obstetrics
The Johns Hopkins University School of Medicine

G. C. A. ANDERSON

Attorney for the Medical and Chirurgical Faculty of Maryland
Former President, Maryland Bar Association

GLORIA BEAN

Clinical Social Worker, Woman's Clinic, The Johns Hopkins Hospital

LONNIE S. BURNETT, M.D.

Assistant Professor of Gynecology and Obstetrics
The Johns Hopkins University School of Medicine

ROBERT C. COOK

President, Population Reference Bureau, Inc., Washington, D.C.

IRVIN M. CUSHNER, M.D.

Assistant Professor of Gynecology and Obstetrics
The Johns Hopkins University School of Medicine

HUGH J. DAVIS, M.D.

Assistant Professor of Gynecology and Obstetrics
The Johns Hopkins University School of Medicine
Director of the Contraceptive Clinic
The Johns Hopkins Hospital

Participants

LEON EISENBERG, M.D.
Professor of Child Psychiatry
The Johns Hopkins University School of Medicine

ELI FRANK, JR.
Attorney
President, Baltimore City School Board

GHISLAINE GODENNE, M.D.
Assistant Professor of Pediatrics
Assistant Professor of Psychiatry
The Johns Hopkins University School of Medicine
Psychiatrist-in-Charge, Adolescent Service
The Johns Hopkins Hospital

ETHEL M. NASH
Assistant Professor of Preventive Medicine
Associate in Obstetrics and Gynecology
The Bowman Gray School of Medicine
Winston-Salem, North Carolina

CLIFTON R. READ
Vice President for Public Education and Information
The American Cancer Society, New York, N.Y.

JOHN ROMANO, M.D.
Professor and Chairman of the Department of Psychiatry
University of Rochester, School of Medicine and Dentistry
Psychiatrist-in-Chief, Strong Memorial Hospital
Rochester, New York

CARL E. TAYLOR, M.D.
Professor of Public Health Administration—
International Health Studies
The Johns Hopkins University
School of Hygiene and Public Health

CONTENTS

Contents

INTRODUCTION

By an historic accident we have come in this decade to the intersection of two paths—the pathway being followed by gynecology and obstetrics as it has grown and developed as a medical discipline and the pathway being followed by our society as it has addressed itself to examining the cause and cure of our threats and ills. At this intersection it has become evident that many of the problems which seriously concern our society are related to the discipline of gynecology and obstetrics. This is not to say that the gynecologist-obstetrician can solve these problems alone, but neither can he hide from them. Our society is asking for help and many of the weapons which are needed are to be found largely in the therapeutic armamentarium of this specialty.

We did not ask for this—we did not seek it out. Nevertheless, we find ourselves at such a crossroads and we cannot flee the responsibility it implies.

The fact that the present conference focuses on the social responsibility of gynecology and obstetrics, however, is not meant to imply that we feel that this is the only area of medical practice which carries such a responsibility.

This discipline is neither so blind nor so chauvinistic as to believe that this obligation is ours exclusively. All of medicine carries a responsibility to the community it serves, and the standards of medical care—the quality as well as the quantity—are not the concern of the physician exclusively; these are the proper business of the people.

By the very nature of its content, gynecology and obstetrics carries perhaps a greater responsibility for a social conscience than do other disciplines, and the evidence for the truth of this statement is on all hands. In the first place, the laws of our various states contain more regulations pertaining to the therapeutic activities usually considered obstetric or gynecologic than there are regulations concerning any other individual branch of medical practice. The legislator who would never dream of promulgating laws about what type of insulin may be prescribed for a diabetic patient will solemnly debate and, indeed, vote for a regulation which proscribes the individualized use of the therapeutic weapons employed by the gynecologist-obstetrician.

In the second place, the profession itself sets aside, and regards with awe, our medical activities. Thus, for example, it is a requirement of the National Hospital Accreditation Commission that there be a staff consultation obtained before every hysterectomy is performed, whereas there is no similar regulation prior to performing a total gastrectomy. In The Johns Hopkins Hospital, as another example, there are listed those operative procedures which are to be the subject of special scrutiny at our regular review meetings. Included on this list is "Every operation on the reproductive tract." I would presume that the hospital administration does not relish the thought of ill-advised or unnecessary gall-bladder operations being performed in this hospital; yet all one can determine from the published regulations is that our department is to review carefully all of its surgery, whereas the general surgeons need review with as great care only a small fraction of theirs.

Finally, our patients themselves provide us with an index of our social responsibility. Seeing us deal in our daily work with the biology of sex and reproduction, it is inevitable that they should bring first to us other problems—the personal and social problems—which refer to sex and reproduction. The girl who encounters difficulties in her marital adjustment is most apt to bring these first to the physician who gave her premarital advice—her gynecologist. The woman burdened by a seemingly uncontrollable sequence of annual pregnancies brings her fears and difficulties first to her obstetrician.

All of these are evidences that we have in truth a different social responsibility than do other areas of medical practice. And these evidences are, in turn, only symptoms of the fact that each of us regards the reproductive tract differently than we regard other parts of the body. The gall bladder is not, in most women's minds, the equivalent of her uterus. We are all quite sure that illness here, malfunction of this part of our lives will have a more profound effect on us, on our family and, multiplying the families sufficiently, on the community, than will malfunctions of our knees, our ears, or other portions of our anatomy.

Introduction

The content of the discipline makes the difference, but, again, gynecology and obstetrics is neither so blind nor so chauvinistic as to maintain that we discharge this obligation alone. It is a responsibility we share with many others: with other departments of the medical faculty, with the social service department, with community agencies, with the schools. To representatives of these several groups, and to others, we have turned for assistance in the presentation of today's panel. Their participation is gratefully acknowledged by all of us, as is their continuing work in these areas of common concern.

We are jointly to consider some of the points at which the science of gynecology and obstetrics impinges most closely on the needs and problems of our society. Consider them and discuss them without being so innocent as to think we can solve all, or, indeed, perhaps any of them. But recognition and delineation is the first step in approaching the solution to any of our problems. Delineation, and the acknowledgment that these are indeed *our* problems. These are not areas for the lawmaker or for somebody else to be exclusively concerned with. They rest near the core of the traditional subject matter of our specialty. As such they are our concern, our interest, but above all our responsibility.—A.C.B.

The Quantity of The Next Generation

THE POPULATION EXPLOSION

The first of the subjects with which we are concerned is the quantity of the next generation, or the population explosion. This problem has been created by a variety of factors, but chiefly perhaps by the sharp decline, within this century, in perinatal mortality. However, what caused a particular disease or problem—where it came from—is never as important as where it is going and what we are going to do about it.

The magnitude of this particular problem almost defies description. Within a few hundred years every man, woman, and child on the face of this earth will have one square yard to occupy. Do not ask, in a cynical or callous way, for war to save the situation. War, over the centuries, has notoriously been a poor way of reducing the population. Indeed, the required remedy must be so much more drastic than warfare that it is entirely possible that whatever we do now will be too little and too late.

There is but one further comment I wish to make. As

1

one who has devoted his life to academic effort, I have a strong feeling about the role of the universities in our society. For centuries these were the repositories of learning, the source of intellectual leadership; from the halls of univeristies came the thoughtful word on social problems. We have witnessed within the past thirty years the formula of the many faculty members who have become governmental advisers; who have created, to a great extent, much of present society.

What I am expressing is a deep personal conviction that when a problem becomes a major one for our society, then it is imperative that the universities address themselves to it. The perfectly evident threat of a drastic overcrowding of our countries and of our globe is of such magnitude, such importance, that it should have priority rating in university centers. Professors of biology, physiology, medicine, and gynecology and obstetrics should be making every effort to provide knowledge and leadership to meet this danger. The university is not an island unto itself—it is a servant of the public good, a leader rather than a follower in intellectual matters. It is fitting that this conference be convening in a university setting, because society's problems are the prime concern of the university. Whether or not this fact is always recognized, whether or not the opportunity is always grasped, the problems of our society must be and must remain a university's major concern.

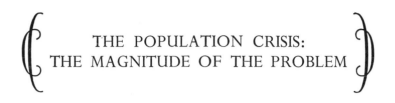

THE POPULATION CRISIS: THE MAGNITUDE OF THE PROBLEM

BY ROBERT C. COOK

The forebrain represents the unique evolutionary innovation which our species, *homo sapiens,* has contributed to the evolution experiment. Slowly, hesitantly, shaken by terror, humankind has gained an understanding of the nature of the universe, of energy, of matter, and of life that apparently no other organism on this planet has ever achieved. The pre-cerebral phase goes back perhaps two million years, with little progress for the first ten thousand centuries. The essential facts about the earth and the solar system and the beginnings of a perspective on man's place in the world of ecology began to be discussed less than four centuries ago.

In this intellectual and conceptual awakening which made the modern world, organized scientific investigation of the facts of life came last. Priests and magicians attempted for two million years to contend with the elemental forces of birth and death and made a mess of it.

3

The key to the causes and control of the epidemic and infectious killers was discovered only about a century and a half ago; effective means to control fertility came later.

I need not review the fantastic results of this tremendous revolution—certainly one of the greatest cultural achievements of mankind, ranking above the discovery of the use of fire, of the alphabet, of agriculture, and the other important breakthroughs—using that term in the anthropological sense.

Man's latent beginnings in playing God by tinkering effectively with those basic elements of the human experience—birth and death—opened up a new era which was called "The Vital Revolution" by the late Norman Himes.

The essential facts of these developments are well known. The age-long, seesaw balance between many births and many deaths, which had held population growth in check since the beginning of time, suddenly changed and the effect has been fantastic. It took a couple of million years for world population slowly and hesitantly to edge up to a quarter of a billion about the beginning of the Christian Era—to double to a half billion took some sixteen centuries. By 1850, world population doubled again to 1 billion and since then has tripled. The current world total, estimated by the United Nations to be 3.4 billion, is expected at least to double by the end of the century to between 6 and 7 billion.

At the present time, there are about 130 million births a year in the world and about 60 million deaths. The net annual gain in population—the difference between births and deaths—amounts to about 70 million. This represents a 2 per cent annual increase.

Without question, the fantastic advances which have been made in the postponement of death rank among the greatest blessings the human race has ever devised. Yet, in the total ecological context on this planet, this runaway increase in numbers of people poses tremendous problems and presents one of the greatest challenges the human species has ever faced.

Population dynamics are simple enough. The balance between births and deaths determines the rate of population growth. There are technical refinements concerned with age distribution and other matters which, though important, do not alter the basic facts. Throughout history the balance has been precarious because mortality has been so high. A balancing high fertility was essential to prevent extinction. Human fecundity during most of man's experience on earth has stood near the physiological limit as an essential element of survival.

Because we are predominantly a uniparous species with a long gestation period, our fertility is modest compared with that of a good many of our mammalian cousins. The birth rate—the number of births per 1,000 population a year—can hardly exceed 60. The ultimate limit of the death rate is over sixteen times as great. In 1348, it is believed that a quarter of the population of Europe died. That would give a death rate of 250. The ceiling on the death rate—namely, 1,000—would occur only once—the year of the bombs when the grisly resources of overkill, now in the launching silos, were exercised to the limit.

So much for background. Now, let us consider the current situation and survey the essential steps to check this alarming growth in world population.

At the present time, the human species splits about two-to-one in its basic demographic pattern. In the Western industrial countries where mortality control first—and very gradually—became effective, a compensatory decline in the birth rate spontaneously took place. In this country, hardly more than a century ago, women were averaging about eight children apiece. This compares with about three at the present time. The reduction in fertility of nearly two-thirds was achieved without any organized planning at any level. Birth control became an issue about 1920, at a time when U.S. fertility was not far from the point of balance with sharply declining mortality.

This same pattern of spontaneous transition is found in all of the industrial countries of the West and very recently in Japan. It is beginning to extend to a few minor enclaves on the edge of mainland Asia. It has not extended to the Asian mainland, to Africa, or to tropical Latin America. In these three areas about 2 billion people—two-thirds of the world's population—still maintain the traditional level of fertility with birth rates ranging upward from 40 to 55.

With sharply declining death rates, the ancient balance between births and deaths is upset with a consequent acceleration in the annual net rate of growth which ranges upward from 2 per cent to 3 per cent, 3.5 per cent, even 4 per cent or more. The death rate is still declining and the current rate of world population increase, namely, 2 per cent a year, still trends upward: it has more than doubled in the past fifty years. This explosive population growth is occurring today in precisely those parts of the world with low standards of living, with marginal diets, and with low levels of literacy.

It is hardly necessary to spell out the gravity of the situation. Hunger is endemic for more than half the human race today, and the threat of famine is very real in large areas of Asia, Africa, and Latin America. The Director-General of FAO (Food and Agricultural Organization), has recently reported that the food production of the world is not keeping pace with the population growth.

Nor is hunger the only problem such rapid population growth engenders. One of the alarming by-products of the reduction of mortality with unchecked fertility is that the proportion of children and adolescents in the population rises very rapidly. In the developing countries today, between 40 and 45 per cent of the population is under fifteen years of age. This compares with 30 per cent in the United States and about 20 per cent in the European countries. The heavy demands for "social capital" necessary to feed, clothe and educate—usually inadequately—these growing hordes of children absorbs much of the hard-won capital these countries are able to generate.

Because of the profound psychoemotional, traditional, and moral imperatives surrounding sexual matters, the problem of reducing fertility to balance steadily declining mortality is extremely difficult. The traditional pattern of high fertility was essential to survival until very recently, and attitudes and customs regarding fertility change slowly.

7

This situation no doubt existed in Europe prior to 1800, but with a slowly declining death rate, time permitted a spontaneous balance between births and deaths to take place without any overt action on the part of governments or private agencies. It took eighty years to drop the death rate in Sweden from 20 to 14. But the timing in the countries in trouble today is very different. In Ceylon, in 1947, the death rate dropped from 20 to 14 *in one year*, eighty times as rapidly as the decline in Sweden. Equally dramatic declines in mortality have taken place in other developing countries. The birth rates have remained high, and no social, political, or religious force now exists which is acting to reduce fertility. The imbalance in births and deaths continues to widen as increasingly sophisticated techniques of mortality control are developed and applied.

The world problem is encompassed in those 130 million births and 60 million deaths each year. To achieve a reduction in population growth that will begin to make possible an orderly development in the cultures of the countries now in demographic stress means that it will be necessary to reduce the numbers of births in the world by some 20 to 40 million a year. Even if the number of births were reduced thus drastically, an excess of 30 to 50 million births would remain.

How is this reduction to be achieved in the heightened demographic tempo of the 1960's? Very frankly, no one knows.

The over-all attack on this surpassingly important problem must be broadly based. Striking improvements have been made in contraceptive techniques, and new techniques have been developed; notably, the now much publicized IUCD (intrauterine contraceptive device). It appears to be working excellently in Taiwan and in other experimental areas. These successes have occurred with populations that are culturally and economically more advanced and somewhat more sophisticated than the massive populations of mainland Asia, of Africa and, to a considerable extent, of Latin America. Not only must the contraceptives be developed and tested and proved to be effective in the most varied social and cultural contexts, but means must be found to "sell" them to the people of these countries. Since this whole population question is obviously right in the middle of that area of emotional turmoil centered around sex, it is obvious that very sophisticated techniques will be needed to carry this essential message to at least a billion Garcias around the world.

There is not, at the present time, any comprehensive plan for dealing with this question. The work that is being done in Taiwan and in South Korea by The Population Council, and the work which is being done by the Ford Foundation in India and Pakistan and other efforts now being initiated by the governments of these and other countries—these are all first steps which are of the greatest importance. But, in terms of reducing the number of births in the world by 20 to 40 million, these efforts must be rated as preliminary pilot studies rather than as even marginally effective action programs.

There are grave questions here of magnitude and of timing. The Director of the Harvard Center for Population Studies—who has had a notable career as an oceanographer of distinction—stated recently that the "population growth problem is not a problem that has to be solved next year. We perhaps have one or two generations before it becomes hopeless. Sooner or later, if rates of population growth continue, one would imagine that the situation would become hopeless, that human beings would be unable to have any hope of controlling their future destiny, but that is not so right now and it may not be true for the next 50 to 100 years. We have some time to work on the problem. It is characteristic of problems that universities and scientists tackle that you must have some time to turn around in."

Ten years ago, a distinguished mathematician and physicist—Dr. Vannevar Bush—warned that the world was even then on a collision course demographically. "But, wars aside, man is still headed for trouble. The world's population is increasing at a rate which renders distress, famine and disintegration inevitable unless we can learn to hold our numbers within reason."

Perhaps the difference in outlook is due to the fact that oceanographers do not have to give too much thought to acceleration, dealing as they do with a rather viscous medium. A simple example will illustrate the situation. If you jump off the front porch, you will likely land all in one piece—with a sprained ankle at worst. Jump off the roof and it is a different story. It is "hopeless" to become concerned over the acceleration by the time you pass the dining room window enroute to the pavement. To imply that we can wait a generation before effective operations adequately begin to be planned is essentially a counsel of despair.

The essence of the population crisis is that when things become "hopeless," it is definitely too late to stop the chain reaction whose end-point is disaster and disintegration.

Effective de-fusing of a 3 per cent increase has to begin at least a generation—better, two generations—before this end-point is reached. The point-of-demographic-no-return is not a generation or so in the future. It is very near—almost certainly before 1970.

In recent years it is true that encouraging developments have taken place. The United Nations has finally begun to move. The United States stands on the threshold of a new and affirmative population policy at home and around the world. As noted above, several of the great foundations have begun to center major efforts in this area. Admirable beginnings have been made in research in contraceptive physiology and techniques—in developing understanding which must precede affirmative action. These and other pilot efforts, which cannot be listed here, are admirable as prelude to what now must be undertaken.

What has taken place up to now must be recognized as no more than a token of what must be accomplished in the face of the ticking clock if the verdict of history is not to be "so very little and so hopelessly late."

In summary—the world picture is ominous. The billion people in the "have" industrial countries have effected their "vital revolution." With low birth rates and controlled birth rates, their rate of growth is moderate. Economic pressures can be expected to reduce further the birth rate if the shoe begins to pinch. This may be happening even in our own most favored country, where the fertility indices have been moving down persistently for nearly two years in the face of generally favorable conditions laced with grave social and economic problems.

The two billion or more people in the "have not"—or "have very little" areas—are currently stuck halfway into the "new vital era." Death rates are starting down and are continuing to decline. Birth rates remain traditionally high. With marginal existence, with endemic hunger, with nascent famine in growing areas, with an increasing burden of populations nearly half children, the situation ranges from bad to desperate—and it is not tending to improve.

It is in this sector that 85 per cent of the projected population increase between now and 2000 A.D. is expected to take place. The situation borders on the desperate. It is hair-triggered to explode into disaster in large areas. Recent FAO surveys show Kwashiorkor—a devastating protein-deficiency disease—existing all over southeast Asia, three-quarters of inhabited Africa, and nine-tenths and more of Latin America. This is only one index of the range, the magnitude, and the gravity of the problem.

It is no exaggeration to say its solution represents perhaps the greatest, the most urgent, and the most complicated undertaking upon which the human race ever embarked. Too little and too late in mounting and pushing the attack spells an inevitable global disaster.

The magnitude of the problem can be expressed in just

one sentence: The current rate of increase, centering in the "have-too-little" countries, must be checked by the *prevention of from 20 to 40 million births a year.*

The oceanographer is on solid ground in holding that this cannot be accomplished next year, nor the year after. Unless substantial progress in reducing world fertility is shown within the next ten years, the outlook borders on the hopeless.

Obviously this is an enormous undertaking. There is a smug assumption going the rounds that tucked away somewhere in the United States is a "solution" which only has to be declassified to save the world. No such magic formula exists.

What does exist—and what is the basis for guarded optimism once the paralysis of too little and too late is overcome—is that substantial beginnings toward a solution are in progress. Fine work in various areas is being done, and this can serve as the launching pad for an accelerated program.

Pushed hard enough, science and dedication can produce virtual miracles with very little time to "turn around." A classic example is the Manhattan Project. The key to the operation of unlocking of atomic energy would have been found in the leisurely tempo of research in the laboratory in due time. Two aging men—one in Washington and one in London—with the power to enlist the necessary resources got the job done in a couple of years. They drafted the best minds in all the free world. It took research and inspiration and daring improvization. The job got done. That it was at great cost is irrelevant.

To say that the number of births in the world cannot be reduced significantly by 1970–75 is a counsel of despair. To say that this will happen in the still relaxed and alarmingly lackadaisical tempo of the over-all operation now emerging is to engage in dangerous make-believe.

That is the problem. Its magnitude is gargantuan. My assignment was to put this in perspective. How the job is to be done is another matter, and to this question I do not have an answer. Nor, I suspect, does anybody else. This can be said: The cloth which is being stitched together today will make a suit which might fit a dwarf. The tailoring required here must clothe a giant.

That the problem is insoluble, I refuse to admit. The people of the United States have accepted a commitment to put a man on the moon by 1970. The dollar cost of this may run to $20 billion. The genius being expended is impressive. If it is deemed by the peoples of this and other nations that it is worthwhile to commit the human race to making Operation Birth-Balance come to pass in the face of the ticking clock, it can be done. Whether it will be done is another matter. Perhaps the operation will cost less in brains, dedication, and resources than putting a man on the moon. If it succeeded and cost twice as much, it would be one of the best investments mankind ever made in his evolutionary adventure.

EVALUATION OF CONTRACEPTIVE
TECHNIQUES FOR DEMOGRAPHIC
POPULATION CONTROL*

BY HUGH J. DAVIS

The magnitude of the problem posed by the population explosion is of such overwhelming proportions that there is virtually universal agreement on the necessity for contraception. While the planned pregnancy cannot be regarded either medically or socially as a disease, the unwanted pregnancy is certainly the world's commonest ill. Political man and theological man have agreed on the necessity for action to relieve the mounting pressure of unwanted children arriving in a world unprepared to receive them. Medical man must now provide effective remedies.

Population control is a matter of such compelling import that it becomes a public responsibility. The American Public Health Association[1] adopted the following resolution in October, 1964: "that Federal, state and local governments include family planning as an integral part of their health program, making funds and personnel available for this purpose, as well as ensuring such freedom

* This investigation was supported by The Baker Fund.

15

of choice of methods, that persons of all faiths have equal opportunities to exercise their choice without offense to their consciences."

It is within the province of the medical profession to examine available methods and determine to what extent they fulfil the criteria of a safe and effective contraceptive. The perfect contraceptive should be absolutely effective, absolutely reversible, psychologically acceptable, theologically acceptable, and totally free of medical complications. There is no such method. But we do have effective contraceptives. It is the purpose of this paper to present the preliminary experience at The Johns Hopkins Hospital with one such method—the intrauterine contraceptive.

Background

Until very recently, even an approximation of an effective contraceptive, psychologically and theologically acceptable, was nonexistent. To be psychologically acceptable in a broad sense a contraceptive must not interfere with the sexual gratification of either partner. The high motivation required for successful use of the diaphragm, condom, and the various jellies and foams applied precoitally has been a major block to effective population control.

While the upper socioeconomic tenth of the population can and does indulge in elaborate precoital rituals to control their fecundity, the lowest socioeconomic tenth rejects such methods. This has been true since the time of the Pharaohs. Cleopatra is said to have uesd a vinegar-soaked sponge in the vaginal vault as a contraceptive. The fellahin, both ancient and modern, have had little interest in chemical and mechanical contraceptives. The birth rate in the city of Baltimore in 1960 reflects this fact: There were 73 births per 1,000 white females in the highest economic class aged fifteen to forty-four, while in the lowest economic class there were 133 births. Thus, the segment of the population least able to discharge the responsibilities of parenthood was producing twice as many children per annum. The difference was nearly triple in the comparable nonwhite group.

Hence the importance attached to two methods which are more broadly acceptable: the pill and the intrauterine device. These methods have been highly effective and reversible, approaching 100 per cent. Their use is remote from the coital act, making them psychologically more acceptable than traditional techniques. Both methods are the subject of continuing medical discussion as to comparative effectiveness and indications, and as to the incidence of significant complications.

The pill has been linked to a small but disturbing incidence of thromboembolic phenomena and strokes, as well as a variety of minor side effects. Medical assessment of the pill must balance the risks associated with its chronic use against the risks associated with a chronic state of pregnancy. Viewed in this perspective, it must be admitted that the rarity of serious complications is such that the use of the pill can be justified. But this is true in a conservative sense only in circumstances which preclude the use of techniques of superior safety. Experience with the intrauterine device has been more limited, hence absolute assessment of medical risks is as yet incomplete.

Ethical Considerations

From an ethical point of view, the pill and the intrauterine device are also the subject of continuing discussion. The fact that they represent new contraceptive techniques, and that their probable mechanism of action differs from that of traditional techniques, raises ethical questions as well as medical questions. Anovulatory medication interferes with the natural process of ovulation, while the intrauterine devices appear to accelerate the natural process of ovum transport, physiologically preventing conception. In the case of the pill, we are preventing conception by delaying ovum release, while in the case of the device, we are accelerating ovum transport. The ethical problems involved are subtle.

Can the pill or the intrauterine device be condemned as abortifacients? I think not. According to the *Encyclopaedia Brittanica*, the term abortion refers to the *separation* and expulsion of the contents of the pregnant uterus. The derivation of the word is from the Latin verb *ab-oriri*, the prefix *ab* denoting motion away from a fixed point. Thus, to separate or detach from its origin, or *oriri*, becomes the essential element in distinguishing abortion from contraception. Abortion requires the detachment of an established *conceptus*, an event which cannot occur prior to the nidation of the fertilized ovum.

Furthermore, it appears logically inconsistent, if not

impossible, to make a distinction between the ethical acceptability of methods which prevent conception by precluding successful conjunction of the sperm and the egg, and methods which prevent successful conjunction of the ovum and maternal bed. The means are alterations in normal physiology, and the result—contraception—is identical. The British Council of Churches[2] pondered this question in 1962, concluding that "A distinction must be drawn between biological life and human life, and that in the absence of more precise knowledge, nidation may most conveniently be considered to be the point at which the former becomes the latter." In this mature perspective both contraovulatory and contranidatory agents are ethically and medically acceptable contraceptives.

General Policies

Experience with the use of the oral contraceptives at The Johns Hopkins Hospital has been limited because of a reluctance to assume medical responsibility for the occasional serious complication associated with the method. But there are other reasons. Patients tend to fall into two broad classes economically and motivationally. Those economically able to afford the continuing cost of oral contraceptives, and motivationally able to keep rigid dosage schedules day-after-day and month-after-month are but a fraction of the candidates for family planning services. Even when the pill is provided gratis in an intensively supervised research program, Rovinsky[3] found that 40 per cent of the initial acceptors in the low socioeconomic group abandoned the method in a few months. And in the field of demographic population control, it is clear that when the cost of the pill approaches the annual per capita income, as in India, the oral method is economically impossible.

For these reasons, the Department of Gynecology and Obstetrics undertook a controlled evaluation of the acceptability, effectiveness, and complications associated with the intrauterine device. Though not the sole method offered to the clinic population, the convenience of the Incon is such that the acceptance rate has been high. A geometric rise in the rate of insertions has been observed as satisfied users refer other women for contraceptive consultation.

Materials and Methods

The intrauterine contraceptive has been offered to parous women, with normal pelvic examination and negative Papanicolaou smear, who express a preference for the method at their six weeks' post partum examination (Fig. 1). Candidates for insertion have been placed on oral contraception (Ortho-Novum 2 mg.) for twenty to forty days, the medication being withdrawn five days prior to the scheduled insertion. By following this plan, most complaints of postinsertion bleeding have been avoided since the patients are already menstruating. Second, insertions in the face of clinically occult pregnancies have been avoided. And third, it has been possible to schedule insertions efficiently in a weekly clinic under skilled supervision.

The intrauterine device which has had significant evalua-

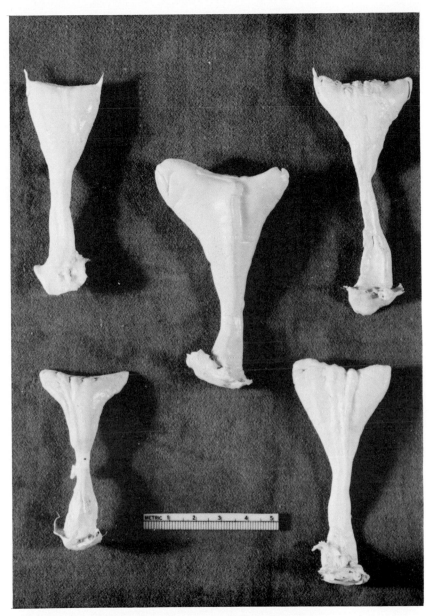

FIGURE 1. Silicone rubber molds prepared from vaginal hysterectomy specimens, illustrating variations in normal uterine size and configuration. All five specimens are from parous women, four to six months post partum.

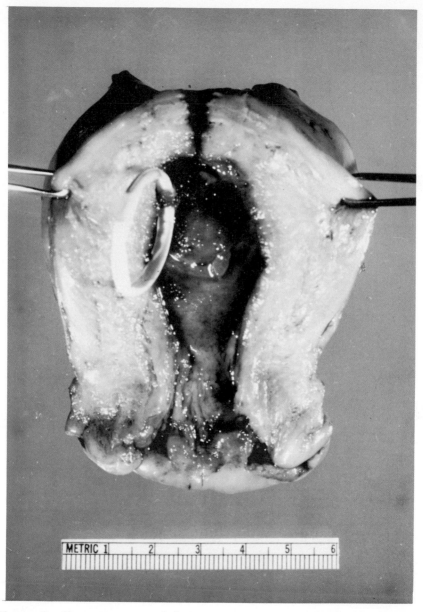

FIGURE 2. Gross appearance of the uterine cavity six months after insertion of Incon. Patient had moderate bleeding for three days post-insertion, normal menses thereafter. Grooving of endometrium evident where ring was seated.

tion in the department of gynecology and obstetrics at Johns Hopkins is a simple closed ring-design molded of ultrathene, a chemically inert plastic with superior recoil characteristics. The diameter of the open ring is 25 mm., corresponding to the mid-range of uterine cavity sizes reported in a previous publication.[4] To confirm the presence of the device during follow-up examinations, a monofilament of 0-0-0 blue nylon was securely tied to the ring and allowed to present 3 cms. at the external cervical os (Fig. 2). Insertions were carried out with a modified uterine polyp forceps which compresses the ring to a closed transverse diameter of 6 mm. The ring has an A-P diameter of 3.5 mm. No dilatation is required because the internal os is oval in contour. Routine follow-up examinations were made at two months, six months, and twelve months postinsertion.

Incon Results

Experience, to date, with the Hopkins intrauterine contraceptive can be summarized as follows:

Insertions to March 1, 1965	403
Pregnancies observed	1
Indicated removals	4
Primary expulsions observed	20
Secondary expulsions	10

It is apparent that 388 of 403 women are carrying the device and are free of significant medical complications at this time. Net effectiveness in terms of continuous use is

21

Hugh J. Davis

96 per cent. Contraceptive effectiveness in terms of observed pregnancies in continuous users of the Incon is
better than 99 per cent. Expulsions and indicated removals
in persistent menometrorrhagia have been quite low, and
the only notable complication observed was two cases of
endometritis.

The gonococcus was successfully cultivated biologically
from one of these women, so that the role of the Incon in
her infection is hypothetical. Still, there is some additional
evidence of low grade endometrial reaction. Examination
of the Papanicolaou smear six months postinsertion dis-
closes increased numbers of histiocytes in some patients as
compared with preinsertion smears and controls matched
for age, parity, and phase of the menstrual cycle. There is
also a tendency for smears from some Incon wearers to
demonstrate occasional active-appearing metaplastic cells
of endometrial origin. Such atypical findings might well
be reported as suspicious, much as those associated with
trichomonas infestation can be a source of cytohistologic
confusion. No cytologic or histologic evidence of carcino-
genesis, either in the cervix or endometrium, has been observed secondary to fitting with an intrauterine contraceptive. Because of the rarity of significant endometrial reactions to the presence of the Incon, it appears probable
that contraceptive programs will actually act as a cancer
preventive measure by bringing high-risk groups of women
under regular medical control.

Although the preliminary results with the Incon appear
encouraging, it must be stressed that long-term observations may temper our judgment. As with any other contra-

ceptive method, indications for use must be carefully defined if satisfactory results are to be expected. It is not, after all, the only effective contraceptive available.

Summary

1. The mounting social, economic, and medical problems posed by the population explosion demand serious consideration.
2. Political man and theological man are agreed that effective remedies must be applied. The profession must evaluate contraceptive methods with respect to safety and effectiveness.
3. The availability of oral and intrauterine contraceptives provides techniques suitable for broad application. The intrauterine device appears more effective in populations with low motivation.
4. Preliminary results at The Johns Hopkins Hospital indicate that the intrauterine contraceptive may be sufficiently free of significant complications to justify its use in population control.

Reference Notes

1. *American J. Public Health,* **54**: 2101, 1964.
2. British Council of Churches; *Human Reproduction* (London, 1962).
3. Rovinsky, J. J., *Obst. and Gynec.,* **23**: 840–50, 1964.
4. Proceedings of the Second International Conference on Intrauterine Contraceptive Devices. Excerpta Medica International Congress Series (Amsterdam, 1965).

PROBLEMS IN MOTIVATION
IN FAMILY PLANNING

BY CARL E. TAYLOR

The population explosion is producing a popular press explosion. This does not mean, though, that public motivation to use family planning is keeping pace with the number of articles being written. Effective implementation of national family planning programs is crucial to the success of national development programs in many developing countries. Family planning is being included in an increasing number of welfare programs in this country and with the present poverty program such activities will probably increase.

Let me start by presenting briefly some assumptions which should clarify a subsequent discussion of motivation.

The problem of population increase is perhaps the greatest health and social problem of our time. The acuteness of the problem should be particularly evident to practicing doctors who see in individual families the serious consequences of failing to try to adjust the numbers of children to the family's ability to care for them.

The problem is going to get worse regardless of what

we do at this stage. We are caught up in a demographic cycle of development which carries an intrinsic pressure for a major population surge which is essentially unavoidable. This statement is based on the standard demographic finding that the process of development causes both death rates and birth rates to fall. The death rate decline necessarily precedes the fall in birth rate because parents logically will not stop having babies until there is some assurance that those they do have will survive. This historical fact could be illustrated by data from many countries but is summarized in Figure 1 which synthesizes general trends to show the demographic gap, or the lag period, by which the birth rate's fall follows the death rate. During the transitional period, every population on which we have observations has undergone a two- to three-fold increase which has provided the increased manpower for industrialization. In Western countries, the transitional period extended over as much as two centuries. With modern public health techniques we can produce a precipitous fall in the death rate. The big question is whether we can make the birth rate follow the death rate within one or two generations rather than one or two centuries. Like so many things in modern life a social control mechanism that used to be self-regulatory has been thrown out of balance by rapid development in a particular type of activity. When birth rates and death rates both were about 30 to 40 per thousand population, birth rates were relatively stable while death rates fluctuated widely up and down as a result of major epidemics and famines. When both birth rates and death rates drop to the 10 to 20 range

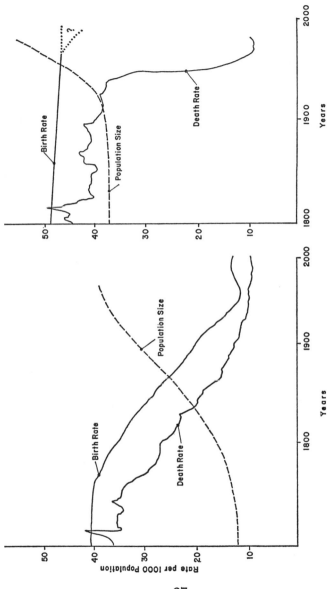

FIGURE 1. (Left) The Demographic Gap and Population Increase in Western Countries. (Right) The Demographic Gap and Population Increase in Developing Countries.

27

the relationship is reversed with death rates now remaining stable while birth rates fluctuate in cycles depending on factors such as economic prosperity, social pressures, and fashion. Birth rates are amenable to change. One other important difference to be noted in the two graphs is the dramatic fact that most developing countries have the disadvantage of starting their development with considerably greater population density than was found in Western countries before their population increase started. Figure 2 shows the marked shift in the balance of world population that is projected for the year 2000.

The specific effect of disease control is shown in Figure 3, giving the size of the population increase between decennial census counts in India.[1] The population increase is even greater since 1961, going up by about 12 million each

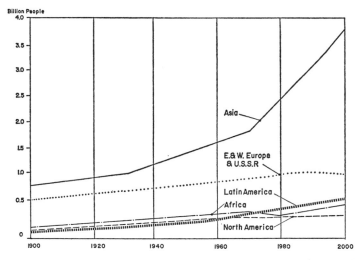

FIGURE 2. Growth of World Population—Geographic Regions, with Projections.

year. The lack of increase in 1871–81 can be attributed to specially severe famines, in 1891–1901 to a severe nation-wide plague epidemic, and in 1911–21 to the 1918 influenza epidemic. The change since 1951 is due to the beginning control of malaria and other endemic diseases, particularly those affecting children.

In this paper we shall concentrate on the population problems of individual families rather than on mass statistics. Put in its simplest terms, the population problem is due to the fact that in any underdeveloped situation, whether overseas or in Baltimore fifty years ago, parents had to have six to eight children in order to raise three

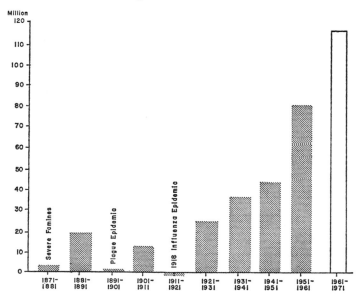

FIGURE 3. Population Increase in India (in millions) by Decennial Periods—1871–1971. (Decade 1961–1971 projected on basis of rate of increase 1961–1965.)

29

or four. Approximately half of all children die before developing immunity to the usual range of pathogenic organisms in their environment and becoming accustomed to an adult diet. With the introduction of relatively simple elements of better living almost anywhere in the world, only occasionally will parents lose a child. To maintain a stable population in a country where the marriage rate is as high as in the U.S. or India the average married couple should have two or occasionally three children. Even if the average completed family size is four or five there will be doubling of the population in every generation.

However, I do not believe that conditions will ever get as bad as is predicted by certain writers who foretell in extravagant terms the mathematical prospects of doom if present uncontrolled fertility continues. For instance, it is possible to demonstrate mathematically that at present rates of increase we will have 1½ sq. feet per person by 2500 A.D. or that in five thousand years the human mass will be reproducing so fast that it will form a solid ball of flesh growing out into space at the speed of light. This type of mathematical exercise is patently ridiculous. Human beings are adaptive and pragmatic. Wherever population pressures have become acute in the past, they have been relieved either through social adjustments or through a deterioration in health conditions. The classical example of social adjustment is the experience of Ireland after the potato famines of the early nineteenth century when the total population was reduced from a high of about 8 million to the present level of about 4 million through emigration. The lower level of population was then maintained by basic changes in inheritance laws and other social pressures which resulted in one-third of women never marrying while those who did marry waited until they were almost thirty years of age. Historically, in several countries, female infanticide was the traditional and a highly effective method of population control. Japan is the classical example of a country which has rapidly and dramatically produced population balance by legalizing abortions.

As a final general statement I would like to stress the complexity of the effort to increase motivation for family planning. One should expect the unpredictable.

Let me turn now to an oversimplified presentation of the complicated interactions which control motivations for family planning. Figure 4 shows a diagrammatic model

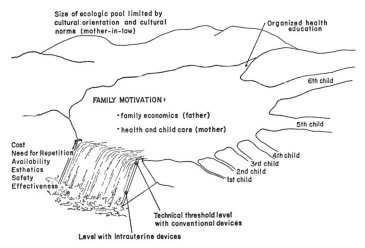

FIGURE 4. Family Decision-Making about Use of Contraception.

illustrating the interactions between some of the more important factors involved.

Family decision-making about birth control can be illustrated by the simple picture of a dam, a pool, and a series of streams flowing into the pool. The dam represents the technical difficulty of using available contraceptive methods and includes such practical elements as availability, cost, esthetic considerations, safety, need for repeatedly remembering, and actual effectiveness in use. The pool represents the parents' combined level of motivation for family planning. When the technical difficulties are great a high level of motivation will be needed. But when methods are easy a low lovel of motivation will flow over the dam into effective use. It is, for example, increasingly evident that motivational levels that would preclude effective use of traditional contraceptives are completely adequate for the intrauterine contraceptive devices. Field studies in Taiwan, Korea, Pakistan, and elsewhere indicate that one feature of the IUCD's is that there is a great deal of woman-to-woman spontaneous spread of information. The bed of the pool can be considered to be the basic cultural orientation toward children of the social group as represented by the stereotype of the mother-in-law's attitudes. If the culture favors large families it will take a lot of motivation to fill the pool. The father's motivation tends to be influenced primarily by family economics and the mother's by the day-to-day problems of child care and the health of family members, including herself. Flowing into the pool are streams of different sizes each representing the birth of a child. A trickling stream starts with the first child. With the births of second and third children, stream size progressively increases. Starting with the fourth child there are even larger streams flowing into the motivational pool with each birth. By the sixth child stream size is usually so large that parents will use extreme measures in meeting technical difficulties. Many surveys in India and elsewhere indicate that parents say that their ideal family size is three-plus children. The difficulty is that they are not willing to do anything about this somewhat vague wish until they are up to five or six children. Where there is a national health education program or readily available private information sources additional streams can be visualized flowing into the pool to build up motivation. The main effect of health education, however, will probably be in providing information about family planning methods and their availability rather than in actually contributing much to building up motivation.

We turn next to more detailed analysis of the factors which directly influence motivation for family planning and what can be done about them.

From the health worker's point of view, the most compelling reason for using contraception is when the mother's health is jeopardized by further pregnancy. Related to this is the well-known secondary effect on the health of children. Textbooks and standard reference carry frequent comments such as the following statement by Dr. Barnes:[2] "age and high parity are associated with many congenital defects, mongolism for one. For women of advanced age, or women who have already had a number of children the importance of using contraceptive techniques as preventive measures should be obvious." I will not try to marshal the evidence for this conclusion because it is very spotty. The extent of the problem can be best illustrated by specific examples from high-risk groups. Meier[3] studied a small group of multiparous women on relief in an urban area and found that one-third of their children were "unwanted" by even the most elementary criteria; one-fifth of the women had serious health hazards prior to their fourth confinement and another two-fifths had serious health hazards after their fourth pregnancy with only the remaining two-fifths having no major health complaints. Due to the hazards of childbirth in many underdeveloped countries the life expectancy of women is significantly lower than that of men. There are up to 20 per cent fewer women surviving through the childbearing period than men.

Direct evidence of deleterious effects of frequent and rapid childbearing on the health of children comes from a long-term study based at Khanna in Ludhiana District in the Punjab.[4] A careful study of the 1,479 children born in eleven Punjab villages and followed for three years, showed a clear-cut relationship between mortality and both the interval between pregnancies and the mother's parity. Table 1 shows a dramatic difference between the mortality of babies born less than two years after a previous pregnancy as compared with those born after an interval of more than two years. Differences in neonatal mortality are most marked, but infant mortality is also highest, after a short interpregnancy interval. Although many factors undoubtedly contribute, an indication that

34

TABLE 1. Mortality of 1,479 Children Born in Eleven Punjab Villages, 1955–58, by Interval between Observed and Preceding Child*

Interval between births in months	Number of births	Neonatal mortality: deaths per 1,000 infants aged less than 28 days (N = 1,479)	Infant mortality: deaths per 1,000 population aged less than 1 year (N = 1,457)	Second year mortality: deaths per 1,000 population (N = 854)
Primip.	231	95.2	175.4	68.7
0–11	34	88.2	205.9	105.3
12–23	432	97.2	201.9	54.9
24–35	491	57.0	132.2	89.0
36–47	175	57.1	137.9	57.7
48+	112	35.7	108.1	29.0
Unknown	4	0.0	0.0	0.0
Total	1479	73.7	160.6	67.9

* Reproduced by Permission of American Journal of the Medical Sciences, 240: 361, 1960.

competition for food and care may be partly responsible is the fact that differences persist into the second year mortality or weaning period. Table 2 relates these same mortality patterns to parity. Other than the high rates of mortality associated with primiparity there is a steady increase in risk associated with increasing parity which is most evident with the second year or weaning period mortality.

The next question, then, is: How important to parents are health implications as compared with other factors such as economic status? In the classical Indianapolis study of middle-class Americans[5] questions were asked about what would be considered valid reasons for using contraception. Ill health was given as an appropriate justification in 58 per cent and poor economic situation in 27 per cent of the group interviewed. Studies in India, Chile, Jamaica, and Puerto Rico also show health to be an important motivational consideration. As an example the results from Hatt's study of over 13,000 adults in Puerto Rico[6] show the balance between health and economic factors in motivating. Although health was accepted as an important reason for limiting family size with 21 per cent of the responses, economic problems were considered even more important, being mentioned by 54 per cent of those interviewed. The relative importance attached to these two factors is approximately reversed in comparison with the Indianapolis study, a finding probably related to the greater poverty in Puerto Rico. In the Punjab study referred to above,[7] the reasons for acceptance of family limitation again showed that twice as many people were influenced by economic considerations

TABLE 2. Mortality of 1,479 Children Born in Eleven Punjab Villages, 1955–58, by Parity* (A Field Trial of Population Control)

Parity	Number of births	Neonatal mortality: deaths per 1,000 infants aged less than 28 days (N = 1,479)	Infant mortality: deaths per 1,000 population aged less than 1 year (N = 1,457)	Second year mortality: deaths per 1,000 population (N = 854)
1	230	95.7	171.8	75.8
2	209	52.6	116.5	15.6
3	210	81.0	144.9	24.2
4	197	30.5	123.7	92.4
5	165	84.8	171.8	95.7
6	136	51.5	164.2	76.9
7–12	326	95.1	206.3	95.0
Unknown	6	166.7	166.7	0.0
Totals	1479	73.7	160.6	67.9

* Reproduced by Permission of American Journal of the Medical Sciences, 240: 361, 1960.

as health. Further analysis of these data showed that when people already had so many children that they were ready to stop completely they usually gave an economic justification. When, however, the parents said they wanted more children but were now interested in spacing births, the reason was more often related to health. This distinction may also apply to the previously noted difference between Puerto Rico and the United States. In many developing countries the general pattern is to have a large family and then stop, while in the more developed countries the concept of spacing is more generally accepted.

Other social factors which directly influence motivation for family planning can be only briefly covered. I will present data drawn from the Indianapolis study[8] but the findings have been confirmed by others. The importance of education has long been recognized. Up to twenty-four years of age, less than 60 per cent of women with only grade school education used contraception while there was a progressive increase of use in the higher educational groups up to over 90 per cent for college women. In older women there was a sharp increase in use of contraception in both college and high school women with percentages of use going up and over 95 per cent but those with only grade school education never went over 80 per cent usage even though they were considered middle class. Lower-class rates of contraception usage are much lower but rather than blaming the women we should attribute this to ignorance and lack of availability. The most important socioeconomic consideration today is the great need for family planning to be made available in families who are indigent and on public welfare and for appropriate health education as part of original maternal and child health programs. It is in this group that a method as simple as the IUCD will make its greatest contribution. The growing movement to make family planning a routine part of welfare services is most encouraging. The number of states which have such programs has gone up from twelve in 1963 to twenty-five in 1965.

Finally let us consider the relationship between the attitude of doctors and the motivation of patients toward family planning. There have been several studies of doctors' attitudes. My data are from a report issued two years ago by Cornish, Ruderman, and Spivack[9] which was based on detailed personal interviews with a stratified sample of physicians from cities, towns, and rural areas. Doctors were asked about the sources of information about family planning in the community. The doctors reported that 58 per cent of women learn about contraception from their friends and only 27 per cent learn from their physicians. Even more specifically approximately half of the doctors never initiate discussion of contraception either in premarital counseling or post partum examinations. Only one-fourth frequently, or almost always, raise the topic. There is, however, a difference between general practitioners and internists on the one hand, and obstetricians and gynecologists on the other, with the latter specialists initiating discussion of contraception in 50 per cent of their premarital counseling interviews. The differences in initiating discussion of contraception according to the religion of both doctors and patients were particularly great. Non-Catholic

Carl E. Taylor

doctors initiated discussions of contraception in 45 per cent of premarital interviews with non-Catholic patients. Catholic doctors initiated the topic in 11 per cent of interviews with non-Catholics and 10 per cent of interviews with Catholics. The effect of religious convictions is also indicated in the responses to the following question, "A severe cardiac case comes in at post partum examination. Her heart condition made for a very difficult pregnancy. She asks to be taught the rhythm method of contraception. How would you handle this case?" Sixty-six per cent of non-Catholic doctors said that they would urge the use of other methods, while 60 per cent of Catholic doctors said they would teach the rhythm method only. On religion, the very strong conclusion that needs to be reiterated is that there is no basic disagreement between religious groups on the desirability of family limitation. The only differences relate to methods to be used and as methods improve these differences, too, should disappear.

My major thesis is that doctors are not now adequately fulfilling their role in educating their patients about contraception. To be particularly stressed are the data which have been presented indicating that doctors themselves said that more than half of their patients find out about contraception from their friends and only about one-fourth learn from their physicians. Half of all doctors never bring up the subject of contraception and another one-fourth only occasionally raise the question as part of premarital counseling or post partum examinations. These are clearly the best times to introduce the concept of child spacing. One of the best indications of the lack of attention to this important area by the medical profession is the dearth of good research information. Even in reference to the effect of health problems of mothers and children on family planning motivation, there is a striking dearth of good data. We must begin to support with evidence the generalizations that have gotten into our textbooks, and thus provide a better basis for health education. It is unrealistic then to expect a high level of motivation from our patients until we as a medical profession are willing to take family planning seriously. As with other social implications of our professional responsibility we should lead, not follow, the important social movements of our time.

Reference Notes

1. Population Reference Bureau, Inc., *Population Bulletin,* 19(1):7, (Feb.) 1963.
2. Barnes, Allan C., *The Johns Hopkins Magazine,* 15(1):10, (Oct.) 1963.
3. Meier, G., "The Effect of Unwanted Pregnancies on the Relief Load," Mimeographed Report, Research Department, Planned Parenthood Federation of America, Inc., June, 1959.
4. Gordon, J. E., Singh, S., and Wyon, J. B., "A Field Study of Deaths and Causes of Deaths in Rural Populations of the Punjab, India." Reprint from *The American Journal of the Medical Sciences,* 241(3), March, 1961.
5. Freedman, R., Whelpton, P. K. and Campbell, A. A., *Family Planning Sterility and Population Growth* (McGraw-Hill, New York, N. Y., 1959), p. 170.
6. Hatt, P. K., *Backgrounds in Human Fertility in Puerto Rico* (Princeton University Press, Princeton, N. J., 1952), Table 60.

7. Gordon, J. E. and Wyon, J. B., "A Field Study of Motivation to Family Planning." Proceedings of the Sixth International Conference on Planned Parenthood, New Delhi, India, Feb., 1959.
8. *Ibid.*, p. 117.
9. Cornish, M. J., Ruderman, F. A., and Spivack, S. S.: "Doctors and Family Planning." National Committee on Maternal Health, Publication No. 19, New York, 1963:19:58.

The Quality of the Next Generation

THE CONCEPT OF FETAL EXCELLENCE

INTRODUCTION

It is entirely possible—indeed probable—that the preceding topic and the one this section deals with are closely related in an inverse fashion. That is to say: one could make a good case for the thesis that some degree of restriction of the quantity of the next generation would automatically produce a considerable improvement in the quality of the next generation. It is certainly true that there are more damaged children—damaged both in a sociologic and a biologic sense—among the children born tenth and eleventh to a family than there are, proportionately, among the children born second and third. A voluntary limitation of childbearing after the second or third pregnancy—implied as being desirable by the previous speakers—would do much to reduce still further maternal mortality and to improve fetal salvage in its broadest sense.

Saying that such restriction of quantity would improve

43

the quality of the next generation is not to say, however, that this is the only line of attack available. Many other things need to be done; much, indeed, is being done.

In 1930 the maternal mortality in this country was alarmingly high, yet by 1950 it had fallen to what has been (perhaps overoptimistically) called "the irreducible minimum." This remarkable accomplishment within the space of two decades can be a source of considerable pride to the obstetrician-gynecologist, and the achievement of this goal occupied most of the energies of the discipline during these twenty years. The weapons which were employed in this effort were primarily an insistence on clinical excellence (the American Board of Obstetrics and Gynecology for the examination and certification of specialists preceded by many years the establishment of corresponding boards in medicine, surgery, and pediatrics) and, secondly, an insistence on public self-criticism (the maternal mortality survey committees' openly reviewing every maternal death on a county or state-wide basis constitutes a model—recently emulated by the anesthesiologists—which could guide other disciplines). But by 1950 it was clear that fetal and neonatal death rates were not responding to this form of attack, and the discipline has, since then, turned increasing attention to this problem.

The record of the past fifteen years' work in this area has been as impressive as that which reduced maternal mortality. Our knowledge of fetal physiology and of those factors which contribute to fetal welfare, and our ability to diagnose and treat the intrauterine patient has increased apace. Short of the ability to manipulate the chromosome, these studies hold the greatest promise of providing us the necessary background to insure neonatal excellence.

During these same years, the behavioral sciences likewise have greatly extended their knowledge and their field. Since all behavior is learned, this is almost by definition a developmental science. Perhaps if, in the utopian future, we can turn over to the behavioral scientists a biologically sound specimen, and they can then apply their newer perceptions and precepts, perhaps at that time we shall be able to guarantee to society "The Quality of the Next Generation."—A.C.B.

THE ORGANIC BASIS

BY LONNIE S. BURNETT

I want to discuss briefly the very provocative subject of the quality of our next generation, in this case quality on an organic level. For my purposes we need only accept the rather obvious fact that the human body does indeed come in more than one quality; therefore, by definition, some bodies are organically inferior to others.

To emphasize my desire to restrict this discussion to the truly organic aspects of quality—that is, the human body as a functioning machine—it might be rewarding to examine very superficially the human machine and its quality aspects as it might be described in a sales manual prepared by Madison Avenue. The super deluxe model or very best quality, has, first of all, a convenient number of arms and legs (two each) and comes with a highly developed communicative and computer system capable of being programed with experiences into a very nice, functional unit called a nervous system, complete with both memory and reasoning. Standard equipment includes a sealed conduit system to distribute fuel, heat, and other

47

essential items, and this is powered by a permanently lubricated pump with quality, nonleaking valves all with a lifetime guarantee. This top quality product comes in two varieties, sort of a matching set; these two varieties, if they co-operate in the correct way, can reproduce themselves, though it should be pointed out that the quality of their offspring varies considerably.

Any appraisal of the role of the gynecologist and obstetrician as related to the organic health of our next generation must first treat our past and present efforts with the "show me" attitude of a skeptic; this one can do very briefly. Those areas to which one might logically turn as playing a role in fetal excellence would include among others premarital counseling, postmarital genetic counseling, contraception, and prenatal care.

I will dispose of these for the most part with the observation that even in those populations where these disciplines have been practiced with a considerable degree of sophistication, the problem of the second class human machine still exists. The fundamental point is that while these special functions have contributed significantly to fetal excellence and will likely continue to do so, they do not fulfill the needs for total success.

If we are truly determined to make available a first-class human body for each newborn of our next generation we must first accept the fact that traditional methods have failed and will continue to fail. We must be willing to abandon tradition when its only merit is conformity, or our conformity must be made to conform to enlightened reason.

The Organic Basis

Whether we accept it or not, the challenge to improve the quality of our next generation is chiefly the responsibility of our discipline. We are now on the threshold of learning to be physicians to the front-end of the life span, the period between conception and birth. It should go without saying, but nevertheless needs to be said, that the potential of the adult is no greater than the potential of the child, and certainly the potential of the child, or newborn, can never exceed that of the fetus or embryo. We cannot allow the quality of our next generation to be dependent upon the quality of our bailing wire, our paste, our needle and thread, and our ingenuity in putting broken pieces back together.

It would be farcical even to suggest, however, that the responsibility for this vast area of human development rests exclusively with the discipline of gynecology and obstetrics. Nevertheless, the *translation* of the accumulated information from all specialities into a population of better fetuses must remain our responsibility. Our concern over the quality of the newborn must of necessity begin not with a positive frog test but with the unfertilized ovum. Our diagnostic efforts cannot stop with the mother but must include the fetus. Such intrauterine diagnosis has indeed already begun and will logically point to intrauterine treatment of the fetus as it already has in several instances of erythroblastosis. These weapons will undoubtedly multiply, and in their multiplication will extend our range in the care and management of our intrauterine patient.

While no single contribution such as this can be expected to solve the entire problem of neonatal quality, I believe the time has come to break step with conformity and accept a concept expressed earlier by Dr. Barnes and others, a concept which recognizes the right of the child to be wellborn. When a given couple chooses to produce a family of three children, should they not have the right to expect the best three children which they are capable of producing? While nature has her own way of rejecting most second-class products of conception, thereby accounting for the great number of early spontaneous abortions, obviously many products escape this quality control mechanism. Today we can frequently identify very early in pregnancy the female who is at high risk to produce a fetus with severe organic malformation, such as the patient who acquires German measles shortly after conception, the female who is subjected to heavy pelvic irradiation during early pregnancy, and the gravid women exposed to certain teratogenic drugs. It is not unreasonable to expect that in the future our ability at early intrauterine diagnosis might include such conditions as phenylketonuria, mongolism, and fibrocystic disease, especially where there is reason to suspect these conditions. Where such information is available, is it not time to present these facts to the couple responsible for this pregnancy, along with a choice? A choice which includes the alternative of electing to substitute this accident of nature, this organically compromised fetus with a whole one? We have invested vast amounts of time, money, and effort in gaining information which will allow us to exercise some control over our destiny and indeed we have succeeded as attested by the increase in the expected life span to seventy-plus years; can we afford to ignore that information where quality of the human organism is concerned? Such a concept translated into practice would require a redefinition of the term "therapeutic abortion" but could begin to reap results even today. More important, it would open the door to whole new horizons of fetal excellence. For instance, the couple with a genetic complement capable of producing either a child with a gross disease defect *or* an organically normal child might some day be given the prerogative of exercising a choice in the quality of their offspring.

The pregnant female armed with information indicating she is carrying a defective product of conception has the right, if not the obligation, to next inquire about the alternatives. These alternatives clearly must include (1) do nothing and allow the pregnancy to continue because of medical indications, that is to say, intervention would endanger the health of the patient; (2) allow the pregnancy to continue not because this is medically indicated but because interruption is repugnant to the physician based on his moral or religious feelings; (3) allow the pregnancy to continue not for medical reasons and not because intervention would be repugnant to the physician but because there is a law prohibiting protective abortion.

The average pregnant patient presenting to the average physician with such a set of circumstances is, I suspect, rarely presented with such a set of alternatives. Instead she is more often presented with a recommended single course of action which more often than not reflects a careful consideration of all pertinent factors *except* the rights of the pregnant female and the newborn. It seems perfectly obvious that when a decision of this magnitude is being made the physician's obligation and the patient's rights make it mandatory that the motivations behind the decision be accurately identified as medical, moral, or legal. The patient is then presented with the freedom already guaranteed the physician, the freedom to express her own moral convictions, or indeed the citizen's freedom to protest an antiquated law. The plea here is for honesty—honesty in conveying to the patient accurately the true basis for the physician's decision that any given pregnancy must proceed to term. Only when this basis is completely seen and acknowledged can we muster the forces to overcome lethargy and truly guarantee the quality of the next generation.

BEHAVIORAL EXCELLENCE

BY LEON EISENBERG

Evolution is an unsentimental taskmaster. Its reward—survival—is offered only to the fittest. Mere numbers impress it not; witness the species that have risen to dominion only to disappear from the face of the earth because superspecialization for temporary advantage had incapacitated them in adapting to geologic change. Evolution's viewpoint is that of eternity and, for all his present increase in numbers, it is by that criterion that man, too, will be judged.

With man, self-consciousness has been added to the laws of biology. It is within man's grasp to foresee the consequences of his multiplication, to consider quality as a greater good than quantity, and to reorder his behavior before the cataclysm. Whether man will, rests upon just such efforts as ours in this conference.

By quantitative criteria, human reproductive and child rearing behavior would appear to be eminently successful. In the last sixty years we have doubled our numbers and in the next forty we are likely to more than double them again. Before we credit this to man's special capacities, let us recall the admonition of Darwin: "There is no exception to the rule that every organic being naturally increases at so high a rate, that if not destroyed, the earth would soon be covered by the progeny of a single pair. Even slow breeding man has doubled in twenty-five years and at this rate, in a few thousand years, there would literally not be standing room for his progeny."[1]

For a statement a century old, we can forgive the factor of ten by which Darwin underestimated the time at which, by the present geometric rate of increase, we should have transformed this planet to a global slum—were it not for the famine, disease, and internecine warfare that will serve to limit us, do we not limit ourselves.

Darwin's rule on the natural rate of increase implies that, since the only species extant will be those that have survived the rigorous test of natural selection, mechanisms to insure reproduction must have been built into the very biologic fiber of each being. The "drive value" or "pleasure" associated with mating guarantees that it will be sought and carried through against the most formidable obstacles. But mere production of progeny does not suffice. The young must be so constructed or so sheltered that they attain the age of reproductive capacity themselves. As the mammalian scale is ascended, the duration and complexity of child rearing increase many-fold, a curious phenomenon in view of the greater risk of their destruction and the social cost to the species in maintaining them. Its explanation lies in the increasing reliance on *learned* (as opposed to *automatic*) coping behaviors, more flexible and thus ultimately more adaptive, but at the price of requiring a longer apprenticeship for their acquisition. Fittingly enough, the prolonged dependence of the primate young upon the adult serves in itself to bind the individual to the group where he assumes his ultimate role as parent and where the chances of his own survival are enhanced; the solitary primate falls to predators.

The complexity of this rearing process has reached its apex in homo sapiens. For reasons, perhaps, of his upright posture and its effect on the pelvic outlet, man's most unique structure, his brain, undergoes the greater part of its growth after birth. Whereas the ratio between adult and neonatal brain weights in other primates is about 1.5, that for man is about 4. The fourfold expansion in mass is only less impressive than the uncountable sprouting of dendrites and proliferation of myriad synapses, all occurring during extrauterine existence when the infant is subject to the vicissitudes of the environment. It is difficult to escape the belief, though an experimental test of the hypothesis is beyond the scope of available methods, that the very structure of the brain is shaped by experience. Certainly, every nuance of behavior is.

In organisms such as the insect or the bird, adaptation has been attained by an exquisite correspondence of the structures and reflexive behaviors of the species to the details of its microenvironment, although even organisms so humble as these must learn—the insect its leaf, the songbird its song. The automaticity of its adaptation is gained at the cost of a narrowing of its range and a vulnerability to uncommon excursions of environmental conditions. Man has given up all but a few of his behavioral automatisms, though he (perhaps unfortunately) carries many of them with him as atavistic remnants. By virtue of his remarkable capacity to learn and unlearn, man has been able to range over the face of the earth and to survive all but the grossest of nature's cataclysms. But this too is at a price. No part of his development is automatic; his young are at the mercy of the care they receive. If that care is full and rich, the result is creativeness and generosity of spirit; if it be mean and poor, the product will be a stunted and distorted mockery of man's nature. For the greatness we may achieve, we must put our survival at hazard; we cannot put aside the chalice that evolution has fashioned for us so painstakingly.

From the standpoint of the numbers game, it is clear not only that we have been producing young in surplus sufficient to more than offset the periodic mass slaughter of war, a form of social behavior unique to man, but also that we have been rearing them well enough to become self-replicating. The salient phrase here is "well enough." What has been "well enough" is almost certainly no longer so. Two changes have occurred in this century which have no precedent in human history and which render traditional modes of behavior as anachronistic as the armor plate of the dinosaur. By shattering the nucleus, we have seized a power so great that we can now destroy our species and perhaps all life on earth; we have attained such multitudinous numbers that merely sustaining present rates of increase in itself places our survival at jeopardy.

Already, population increase in underdeveloped countries is outrunning gains in productivity, rendering present misery ever worse. With passions rising and the thunderbolts of Jove at our command, we shall require a wisdom greater than we have ever displayed if we are to meet evolution's standard. Whether we rear our young "well enough" will now be measured by their success in finding ways, other than wars, to resolve disputes and in learning how to regulate runaway fertility. They must be able to manage the business of living so that it becomes more than death on the installment plan, a regimented lock-step to the grave, but has room in it for compassion, for creativity, for joy. Kind, not number, of offspring is the touchstone.

To agree on this criterion of quality is not to demonstrate that it is attainable. Must our hopes rest on the slender reed of eugenic conservation? If so, how shall we identify the favorable genotype and how insure its selective reproduction, all men demanding the right to reproduce? Or is the behavior of man malleable? Can nurture modify human nature?

I leave the eugenic issues to others more competent than I. I remain dubious that, except for the exclusion of gross heritable defects, it offers much promise given the time constraints within which a solution must be found. Moreover, without denying genetic differences between men, the genotype sets, for the great majority of mankind, very wide limits within which experience molds the decisive phenotype.

This view of environmental shaping of man's nature,

both intellectual and emotional, is by no means general.
Thomas Hobbes stated in the *Leviathan:* "I put for . . . a
general inclination of mankind, a perpetuall and restlesse
desire of Power after Power, that ceaseth only in death. . . .
(This leads) to a time of Warre, where every man is
Enemy to every man . . . no Arts, no Letters, no Society,
and which is worst of all, a continuall feare and danger of
violent death; and the life of man, solitary, poore, nasty,
brutish and short."[2] If Hobbes is to be discounted as being
a political philosopher, consider the bitter pessimism of
Freud: "The very emphasis of the commandment: Thou
Shalt Not Kill, makes it certain that we are descended
from an endlessly long chain of generations of murderers,
whose love of murder was in their blood, as it is perhaps
also in our own. . . . If we are to be judged by our unconscious wishes, we ourselves are nothing but a band of
murderers . . ."[3] "Civilization is perpetually menaced with
disintegration through the primary hostility of men towards
one another. . . . The tendency to aggression is an innate,
independent, instinctual disposition in man . . ."[4] I have
paired Hobbes and Freud to stress that *both* wrote as
political philosophers; Freud's view, though couched in
pseudobiologic terms, is no more a biologic truth than
Spencer's projection of a distorted evolutionism on to
society to justify laissez-faire industrialism:

> The poverty of the incapable, the distresses that come
> upon the imprudent, the starvation of the idle, and those
> shoulderings aside of the weak by the strong . . . are the
> decrees of a large, farseeing benevolence. . . . We must
> call those spurious philanthropists who, to prevent present

misery, would entail greater misery upon future generations. . . . All defenders of the poor law . . . must be
classified among such. The rigorous necessity which,
when allowed to act upon them, becomes so sharp a spur
to the lazy, and so strong a bridle to the random, these
paupers' friends would repeal. . . . Blind to the fact, that
under the natural order of things society is constantly
excreting its unhealthy, imbecile, slow vacillating, faith-
less members, these . . . unthinking men advocate an
interference that not only stops the purifying process,
but even increases the vitiation . . .[5]

But if Hobbes, Spencer, and Freud invoked spurious biologic laws to lend credence to their misanthropic views, we
must admit that Locke and Rousseau had no firmer em-
pirical grounds for their belief in the nobility of primitive
man in a state of nature.

"The State of Nature has a law of Nature to govern it,
which obliges everyone, and reason, which is that law,
teaches all mankind who will but consult it, that being all
equal and independent, no one ought harm another in his
life, health, liberty or possessions."[6]

"While men remain in their primitive independence,
there is no intercourse between them sufficiently settled to
constitute either peace or war; and they are not naturally
enemies. . . ."[7]

The appeal, whether by misanthropist or philanthropist,
to the hypothetical construct of isolated man in a state of
nature in order to determine his "inclination" violates
biological reality; all primates are social animals, with man
the most advanced example. The human brain attained

its present size and, as far as we can tell from endocranial casts, its present configuration some fifty thousand years ago. The behavior of its earliest possessors is lost to the fossil record except insofar as the artistic rather than merely functional shaping of tools and stylized burials attest to the social determination of that behavior. We can gain some insight into the variability of behavior of our paleolithic ancestors by surveying the differences between contemporary stone age cultures like the aborigine, the Amerindian, and the Eskimo—or even between the Indians of the plains and the Pacific Northwest. And with the further evolution of technology and ideology, ever greater and more sophisticated divergences between the behaviors which men exhibit become apparent. Yet there is no evidence to justify the attribution of these cultural differences to the biology of the races who created them; an infant from the most backward if reared among the most advanced at once takes on the behavioral characteristics of his foster, as against his natural, parents. When we contrast groups divided on social class or ethnic axes within a nation, it is true that we may find significant mean differences—on such psychological measures as I.Q. tests— but of equal significance is the enormous variance within groups such that individuals functioning at any given level of competence are found in each group. Further, the attained competence has been shown to vary with experience and to be subject to change by the introduction of new experience.

What is remarkable about human behavior is its variability rather than any supposed constancies; it is the explanation of that variability that constitutes the challenge to the behavioral scientist. All of this can be no more cogently stated than in the words of Helvetius, French philosopher of the Enlightenment, who wrote:

> Two opinions today divide scientists on this subject. One group says, The mind is the effect of a certain kind of temperament and internal organization; but no one has yet been able by any observations to determine the kind of organ, temperament or nurture that produces the mind. This vague assertion, destitute of proofs, is reduced to this statement, The mind is the effect of an unknown cause or an occult quality. . . . Quintillian, Locke, and I myself, say, The inequality of minds is the effect of a known cause, and this cause is the difference of education. . . .
>
> If I could demonstrate that man is indeed but the product of his education, I should undoubtedly have revealed a great truth to the nation. They would then know that they hold within their own hands the instrument of their greatness and their happiness, and that to be happy and powerful is only a matter of perfecting the science of education . . .[8]

If today we would temper the limitless optimism of that statement by a recognition that the extremes of talent are not sufficiently explained by education alone (and would not expect, as did Fourier, that proper universities could produce a nation of Newtons and Shakespeares), we have firmer grounds for the assertion that much of the difference in adaptive behavior between most of mankind is explicable in terms of differences in experience. If we must admit that the evidence is incomplete, we should also agree that the hypothesis is testable and that the mode of its assessment is fully in accord with the democratic principles on which this nation was founded. Let us but resolve to secure for each child as nearly optimal an environment as we can fashion and observe the outcome as he grows into adolescent and adult. If our hypothesis is correct, we shall have created a world in which we shall want to live as well as have to live; if marked interindividual differences persist despite the equality of opportunity, then for the first time we shall have uncovered the thrust of genetic factors and can be guided accordingly. Adoption of the contrary view (that the differences between men are innate), no less an act of faith, must assume either the indifference of the environment or that this is the best of all possible worlds; in so doing, we would act without proof of our beliefs and would condemn ourselves to awaiting salvation through the workings of blind chance.

Our decision, however, should not be based solely upon the grounds of the operational consequences of our choice. There is a preponderance of evidence in favor of the environmental shaping of behavior, based ultimately upon the quite extraordinary plasticity of the mammalian, and in particular the primate, central nervous system. We have not time to examine this evidence *in extenso,* but some brief review of its major outlines is called for. Let us consider, in turn; experimental animal studies on the effects of (a) sensory deprivation (b) experiential impoverishment and (c) early rearing patterns, and human epidemiologic and clinical studies of the effects of (d) restricted and (e) enriched environments.

Nissen has shown for touch and Riesen for vision that total restriction of stimulation in the infant primate results after some months in permanent functional (as well as anatomical) deficits in the corresponding sensory sphere.[9,10] Hubel and Wiesel,[11-13] in a series of elegant studies on the kitten, have demonstrated that the genetically determined encoding of visual information by the neonatal retina is no longer detectable after three months of excluding light from the eye (and have demonstrated a concomitant loss of geniculate cells). For present purposes, these studies may serve to exemplify the dependence of even the primary receptor system upon environmental input for the maintenance, let alone the further development, of its integrity.

When we turn to behavior organized at a higher level of integration, the findings are entirely consistent with the hypothesis that the development of competence requires richness and variety of experience. Even such behaviors as nest-building and protection of the young in the rodent, which do not appear until triggered by hormonal changes, require for their appropriate display prior environmental encounters, with nest-building materials in the one case and the self in the other.[14] Rodents, canines, and primates, reared in bare cages, bereft of manipulanda and of peers, perform poorly on problem-solving tasks and display bizarre patterns of social behavior.[15,16] The apparent regularities in behavioral development which we have so uncritically taken to represent the unfolding of a genetic species-specific code stem from the correspondences between that code and its customary environment. That is, natural selection has acted to shape the potentialities of each organism in relation to the environment it ordinarily will encounter. It is only when we intervene experimentally so as to intercept the environmental regularities that the dependence of inner structure on outer circumstance becomes evident. No amount of experience will enable a cat to use tools or a chimpanzee to talk, but for either cat or chimpanzee to behave in accordance with its kind it requires the experience ordinarily available to it in its habitat.

The care of the young is clearly not a conscious (i.e., planned) process in the animal kingdom (and, all too often, hardly that in the human kingdom); in the sense of formal tutelage, it cannot be said to be taught. On the other hand, that is not to say that it is not learned, for it is dependent upon the sequential acquisition of a hierarchy of social behaviors that prepare the ground for the appearance of care-taking activities, given the hormonal changes and stimulus configurations provided by mating, pregnancy, parturition, and the appearance of the young.[17] Schneirla and Rosenblatt[18] have demonstrated the interdependence of the behaviors of kitten and cat, each stimulating, and stimulated by, the other. What appears so "automatic" or "instinctive" is based upon the precise interdigitation of genetic, nutritional, hormonal, and experiential factors; the developmental consequences of separation are a function of the stage in this process at which it occurs. Harlow[16] has documented the devastating effects of early isolation upon the social behavior of the monkey.

Even so primary a "drive" as sexuality is severely impaired or disrupted in its execution. Finally impregnated and delivered of young, such mothers not only fail to display the ordinary care-taking behaviors but in fact rebuff and injure their infants. It should be noted that the original description of this experimental condition as "maternal deprivation" was quite unwarranted for the deprivation state extended beyond the loss of mothering to the loss of all peer and group interactions. Recent studies indicate that, despite the absence of mothering, infants allowed to interact with other "motherless" infants attain reasonably adequate social adaptation.[19]

In summary, the animal evidence attests to the transactional development of behavioral sequences, each level of function being dependent upon environmental input for the preservation of its integrity and each new functional attainment widening the environmental stimuli to which the organism is potentially capable of responding. Significant restriction in experience leads to marked impairment of competence, in some cases associated with actual tissue change. Experiential enrichment may enable the animal to acquire skills unusual for its wild state but the differences here are less impressive, both because genetic limitations are marked and are so nicely attuned to the traditional environment that the animal functions at a near optimal level. Sensitivity to social control is greatest in the primate as evidenced by the notable variability in the patterns of behavior exhibited by individual colonies of the same species. Primates are capable of imitating innovations initiated by individuals and hence may perpetuate "crazes" over several generations. All of this is at a level many orders of magnitude below that characteristic of human behavior; the animal evidence serves to affirm the profound influence of organism-environment interactions.

The human evidence, if it lacks the elegance and precision of experimental studies, demonstrates, by its very volume and internal consistency, the exquisite sensitivity of the human developmental process to environmental contingencies.[20-22] We cannot undertake here detailed examination of the many studies which have shown a correlation between I.Q., language learning, motivational factors, psychiatric disorders, and academic achievement,

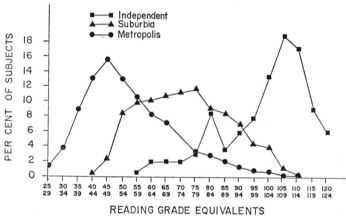

FIGURE 1. Distribution of reading scores, determined by Stanford and Iowa group reading tests, for the sixth grade children in three school populations in 1964 (but excluding classes for the mentally retarded). Number of subjects: Metropolis 12,000; Suburbia 8,000; Independent 200. The figure plots the percentage of the total population reading within each half-year range indicated on the abscissa. Expected mean should be 6.5 (i.e., five months in the sixth grade, the time at which the tests were administered). Metropolis is well behind and Independent well beyond the level.

on the one hand, and social class and ethnic attributes, on the other.[23] Let me, instead, present some data on reading achievement of sixth grade children from four demographic units: "Metropolis," a large American city, "Suburbia," its immediately adjacent county, "Independent," the city's private schools, and "Clinicounty," a bedroom county containing pockets of rural poverty.

Figure 1 plots the first three school populations; it should be noted that it does *not* include the children segregated in classes for the retarded. If this were a plot of heights, one might believe that three different biological groups were here represented. Yet, with the exception of the undoubtedly higher frequency of brain injury stemming from the complications of pregnancy and parturition among the urban poor[24] and of a selective factor governing the independent school intake, these are children that began life with about the same capacities.

Table 1 permits a more quantitative comparison of the reading achievement of the four school populations. Here we see displayed in all its enormity the cumulative consequences of early deprivation, inappropriate and inadequate

TABLE 1. Sixth Grade Reading Levels by School System.

System	Test	% retarded > 2 years.	> 1 year.	% advanced > 2 yrs.
Metropolis	Stan.	28	57	9
Clinicounty	Cali.	15	35	8
Suburbia	Iowa	3	19	34
Independent	Stan.	0	1	82

teaching, and low expectation levels.[25] We have been content to conclude that such data represent a failure of the children rather than a failure of our society and its system of education. School administrators will be quick to point out that the mean I.Q. scores of the three groups are different, as indeed they are, without acknowledging that the I.Q., no less than reading level, is a function of experience. "Metropolis" could not supply figures by race since its records, though not its children, are "integrated." In Clinicounty, however, the percentage of readers retarded by two or more years was three times that for Negro as for white children! Let me add at once that the number of Negro families in social class V was eight times higher than that for whites. The relevant variable here is social class not race; it is an unfortunate fact of contemporary America that race is so highly associated with class.

But perhaps some of you will be inclined to argue that these differences are associated with genotypic factors, the less able being likely to sink to the bottom of the social heap. Against this is the finding that wherever systematic attempts have been made to enrich the educational environment of the child, significant gains in academic attainment and I.Q. have been registered, despite the experimenter's inability to provide these children with an optional total environment. Gray has registered gains in Binet I.Q., Peabody Picture Vocabulary Scores, and Illinois Primary Ability Tests in four year olds after a year of nursery experience.[26] The Higher Horizons Project in New York City has demonstrated equally impressive accomplishments with a total push enrichment at a junior high school level. If these preliminary studies have as yet not obliterated all of the intellectual differences between the impoverished and the advantaged, this constitutes no evidence for an inherent deficit, at least until we have engaged in more massive programs of resuscitation—for it is intellectual resuscitation that is called for—than have so far been attempted.

We confront a curious paradox. Despite the surprisingly general agreement among theorists of widely differing persuasions that early childhood is *the* critical period for moral and intellectual development, formal educational interest in the child does not begin before he reaches six years of age. Yet his first six years have been an epoch of the most rapid changes of his lifetime: tripling of brain size, cytoarchetectonic maturation of all but the phylogenetically most recent brain areas, the acquisition of a sense of self and sexual identity, the elaboration of language, the development of thought and imagination. We have behaved as though we supposed that these remarkable abilities flourish automatically, determined from within by a beneficent providence. Our social consciousness is just beginning to be penetrated by the knowledge that children from impoverished areas are so retarded in these functions that they enter our schools grossly handicapped; hence, our current interest in Project Headstart and other admirable efforts to enrich the beginnings of life. But we have hardly begun to ask: how much more may be possible for the so-called advantaged child if we were to take child-rearing seriously and not assume that, without guidance, mothers "instinctively" know what children need? Forgive the heresy and let me suppose that we were to divert but a fraction of the resources we are willing to lavish upon the race to the moon to the earth-bound study of the process of learning in the child. It is no wild fantasy to suggest that we might well acquire the skill to accelerate intelligence, creativity, and maturity even for this child we so smugly call "advantaged." The argument for the moon race rests upon the grounds that national survival requires it. The argument for the human race seems to me more compelling, for international survival demands it. Let us engage the Russians and Chinese in the competition that matters: the competition for human betterment.

Man, alone of all animals, has the capacity to view his past and to project his future. No less subject than any other living being to the laws of biology, man is unique in his capacity to decipher those laws and to govern his behavior by anticipating their operation. The doctrine of evolution with its basic principle of natural selection is assuredly one of those laws but its meaning has often been misread. Darwin was firm in pointing out: "I use the term Struggle for Existence in a large and metaphorical sense, including dependence of one being on another, and including (which is more important) not only the life of the individual but success in leaving progeny."[27] Whether we shall be successful will depend upon the extent and the degree to which we recognize the importance of endowing each of our children with the resources necessary to become fully human.

The physician who comprehends the significance of

this call has an especial responsibility for mobilizing political action in his community to make it a reality. To some of you, this may seem out of keeping with the traditional role of the physician. Those I would remind of the words of Dr. Benjamin Rush, signer of the Declaration of Independence, a man who remained to serve his patients during the dread Yellow Fever epidemic in Philadelphia when others were fleeing, and, I am proud to add, the first American psychiatrist. In his final lecture to the medical students on the "Duties of a Physician," Dr. Rush recommended:

> a regard to all the interests of your country. The education of a physician gives him a peculiar insight into the principles of many useful arts, and the practice of physic favors his opportunities of doing good, by diffusing knowledge of all kinds . . . in modern times and in free governments, they should disdain an ignoble silence upon public subjects. . . . For the honor of our profession it should be recorded, that some of the most intelligent and useful characters, both in the cabinet and in the field, during the late war, have been physicians.[28]

Let it be said of us that we were among the most intelligent and useful characters, both in the cabinet and in the field, during the war against ignorance, poverty, and overpopulation.

Reference Notes

1. Darwin, C., *On the Origin of Species*, A Facsimile of the First Edition (Harvard University Press, Cambridge, Mass., 1964).
2. Hobbes, T., *Leviathan* (J. M. Dent & Sons, London, 1914).

3. Freud, S., *Reflections on War and Death* (Moffat, Yard & Co., New York, N.Y., 1918).
4. Freud, S., *Civilization and its Discontents* (Hogarth Press, London, 1930).
5. Spencer, H., *Social Statics* (Williams and Norgate, London, 1902).
6. Locke, J., *Two Treatises of Government* (Hafner Publishing Co., New York, N.Y., 1947).
7. Rousseau, J. J., *The Social Contract* (Hafner Publishing Co., New York, N.Y., 1954).
8. Helvetius, C. A., cited in Randall, J. H., *The Making of the Modern Mind* (Riverside Press, Cambridge, Mass., 1940).
9. Nissen, H. W. et al., *Am. J. Psychol.*, **64**: 485, 1951.
10. Riesen, A. H., *Science,* **106**: 107, 1947.
11. Hubel, D. H. and Wiesel, T. N., *J. Neurophysiol.*, **26**: 994, 1963.
12. Wiesel, T. N. and Hubel, D. H., *Ibid.*, **26**: 978, 1963.
13. ———, *Ibid.*, **26**: 1003, 1963.
14. Birch, H., *Am. J. Orthopsychiat.*, **26**: 279, 1956.
15. Thompson, W. R. and Heron, W., *Canad. J. Psychol.*, **8**: 17, 1954.
16. Harlow, H. F., *Am. J. Orthopsychiat.* **30**: 676, 1960.
17. Lehrman, D. S., "Hormonal Regulation of Parental Behavior in Birds and Infrahuman Mammals" in Young, W. C. (ed.), *Sex and Internal Secretion* (Williams and Wilkins, Baltimore, Md., 1961).
18. Schneirla, F. C. and Rosenblatt, J. S., *Am. J. Orthopsychiat.*, **31**: 223, 1961.
19. Harlow, H. F., *Science,* **148**: 666, 1965.
20. Eisenberg, L., *Ann. Rev. Med.*, **13**: 343, 1962.
21. Yarrow, L., *Psychol. Bull.*, **58**: 459, 1961.
22. Deutsch, M., *Am. J. Orthopsychiat.*, **35**: 78, 1965.
23. Passow, A. H., *Education in Depressed Areas* (Columbia University Press, New York, N.Y., 1963).
24. Pasamanick, B. et al., *Am. J. Orthopsychiat.*, **26**: 594, 1956.
25. Eisenberg, L., "Neuropsychiatric Aspects of Reading Retardation," presented at the American Academy of Pediatrics Spring Session, April, 1965.

26. Gray, S. W. and Klaus, R. A., "An Experimental Pre-School Program for Culturally Deprived Children," annual meeting, A.A.A.S., Montreal, December 29, 1964.
27. Darwin, C., *Origin of Species.*
28. Rush B., *Selected Writings* (New York Philosophical Library, 1947).

The
Control of Neoplasia

INTRODUCTION

After beginning in the early part of the century with a
surgical attack on pelvic cancer, the gynecologist moved
during the 1920's to the use of the cauterizing iron, then
to the direct application of sources of radiation, then to the
addition of external irradiation from various modalities,
and finally back to radical surgery. Having come full cycle
under the guise of progress, one fact became apparent from
the results. This experiment in methodology of treatment,
if one chooses to regard it this way, led to the inescapable
conclusion that *the best therapist in the world is limited
by the stage at which the disease is discovered.*

Radium, radioactive cobalt, cancer chemotherapeutic
drugs—all of these are of interest and importance, but
none of them will solve the problem to the same extent
that it may be solved by discovering the malignancy while
it is still incipient. The urgency of this truth has led
gynecologists and obstetricians to adopt and sponsor the
cytologic approach to cancer detection—epitomized most
familiarly in the Papanicolaou cell spread—and to re-
introduce and popularize the concept of carcinoma-*in-situ*,
cancer before it comes cancer.

The public health problem which this presented is well known. To accomplish either a cancer detection cell study or a cervical biopsy, the patient must first come to the gynecologist's office. Since cancer of the uterus, ovary, or cervix are largely asymptomatic lesions, the patient must make this visit to her gynecologist in the absence of symptoms.

To induce patients to do this has not proven easy. Americans are geared to go to the doctor's office armed with specific complaints which will justify the visit. Huge sums of money have been spent—by the physicians themselves, by the American Cancer Society, and by other agencies—to persuade the asymptomatic woman to attend her physician regularly.

In general, however, only two groups of people in our society have accepted the idea of going regularly to a doctor's office without complaints: the pregnant woman, and the mother of a child under the age of one. As soon as these two episodes are over—and they succeed each other in time—women tend to relapse into the comfortable but erroneous concept that only pain, bleeding, discharge, or sterility should take one to the gynecologist's office. When Dr. Hugh Davis introduced his "do-it-yourself" smears, which can be taken at home, among the many inquiries which flowed into the departmental office were letters from physicians pleading for one of the devices so that their own wives, whom they had been unable to persuade to get a check-up, could have some degree of protection against pelvic cancer!

We have long preached two axioms: one, that the detection device for cancer of the breast is the patient herself, and statistically it is true that most women tell their doctors about suspicious breast lesions. On the other hand, the doctor's office is the detection center for pelvic malignancies, and most patients are told by their physician of the existence of this lesion. The second axiom is that no method of diagnosis will protect the woman who stays at home.

The possibility that this second axiom may have been violated somewhat by the introduction of home detection devices in no way alters the fundamental nature of our responsibility in the control of neoplasia. We do not need other ways of burning these tumors more severely, or other techniques of cutting them out more widely; *we need earlier diagnosis.* This, in turn, gives us the responsibility for the instruction of women, for persuading the community that preventive medicine is not something relegated to our health departments but rather something to be practiced in every home of the land; the responsibility, in short, of education for self-preservation.—A.C.B.

EDUCATION FOR PREVENTION*

BY CLIFTON R. READ

Gynecologists have always played an important role in the American Cancer Society—the main drive in 1913 for the formation of the American Cancer Society for the Control of Cancer, our parent organization, came from gynecologists concerned over uterine cancer and their wish to persuade patients to come earlier.

Cancer of the uterus in the United States was for many years a most feared disease. It terrified women and was for physicians, who had to treat it in advanced stages, a frustrating and defeating problem.

In these comments I plan to give a brief historical review of the educational effort of the American Cancer Society to reduce mortality from this type of cancer. As a layman, I will rely very considerably on popular terms and refer to cancer of the uterus, since this is the term we have used in our public education. Though the uterus encom-

* This paper is based in part on one delivered at the Biennial Meeting of the International Union Against Cancer in Mexico City, Feb. 4, 1964.

passes more than the cervix, our feeling was that "cervix" would be less understood than "uterus." Instead of cytological examination, I will usually speak of the Pap (Papanicolaou) smear, or Pap test.

The American Cancer Society cites 1937 as the date of our first truly national public education attack on uterine cancer. That year the Society launched, with the close support of the General Federation of Women's Clubs, what is called the Women's Field Army, seeking particularly to educate women about the danger signals of cancer and the value of the annual checkup.

From the beginning, in public education, the news media have played a significant part. Thus, in 1937, our work was given major impetus by articles in *Life, Time, Fortune,* and a ten-minute filmed review of cancer control in the old "March of Time." These are good examples of journalism with a sense of social responsibility.

What does happen after a magazine or newspaper article on cancer is read? Well, there may be general confusion. I know how difficult it can be to convince a worried relative that newspapers are not the best source of medical information about a particular case. What makes *news* sometimes does not make good medicine.

However, let us assume the article is a sound one, ideally prepared in consultation with a physician. Does a woman read it and rush to her doctor? Sometimes. But books and articles rarely motivate directly, though we do think frank, positive articles about this disease help create a receptive attitude and dispel ignorance and fright. Some fear will always remain—the person who is not afraid of cancer would be foolish—but we believe that people who have read and heard informed discussion about this disease are far more likely to act to relieve their fears by going to a doctor promptly than will those who frown upon cancer education as likely to cause phobias.

The media have another kind of influence: a few months after the first broad national educational effort in 1937 the Congress of the United States established the National Cancer Institute, which was to play such an important part in developing cytology and in the reduction of mortality from uterine cancer.

I wish I could say that the considerable prewar public education effort included what we now know as the "Pap smear." It, of course, did not, since the applicability of this method was not yet sufficiently recognized.

Dr. George N. Papanicolaou, in studying vaginal fluids from ill and normal women, seems to have first noticed cancer cells in 1923.[1] He made a preliminary report in 1928, on which the *New York World* reported: "Discovery of a new method of diagnosing certain kinds of human cancers was announced . . . there is even hope that pre-cancerous conditions may be detected." There was so little interest in his report that Dr. Papanicolaou dropped his research for ten years and then in 1938, in collaboration with Dr. Herbert Traut, began again the work which led to their epochal book, *Diagnosis of Uterine Cancer by Vaginal Smears,* published by the Commonwealth Fund, in 1943.

In 1937, when the Women's Field Army was launched, mortality from uterine cancer was 26.4 per 100,000

81

females; ten years later, it was 22.7 per 100,000 females.[2] There were many factors involved in this significant drop, and one, we believe, was the public education of women.

In 1947 the *Woman's Home Companion* and the *Ladies' Home Journal* each published articles on cytology and cancer. Many regarded these articles as premature, but they were the first major steps in public education in cytology in the detection of cancer, and they led to discussion, letters, debate. Early in 1948 the American Cancer Society sponsored, in Boston, Massachusetts, a meeting of pathologists and cytologists that opened the way to general medical acceptance of the new method. For a number of years the society urged the value of cytology in cancer detection to physicians in conferences, in medical publications, and in films.

The acceptance of this technique has been sporadic; many cities began their own programs relatively early. The American Cancer Society was concerned lest too much enthusiasm develop among women before physicians were ready for them. Thus, in a ten-step society program for our units, the first six steps dealt with the medical profession, with facilities and personnel for interpreting slides. After a community had undertaken these six steps, only then was the seventh, public education, to begin. The society launched its national public education program in 1957, with its film "Time and Two Women," and other material.

While we have always stressed the importance of continuing education to change attitudes toward cancer, with much emphasis on reaching youngsters in their late teens, this particular program has been presented with isolated aggressive thrusts with all the paraphernalia of publicity, and forward drives in particular places, followed by a slackening of peak effort while the surrounding areas caught up.

To mention a few of the cities that have had excellent programs, the earliest was the Toledo and Lucas County program begun in 1947, sponsored by the Academy of Medicine and the American Cancer Society, in which about 105,000 women have been registered, including some women from nearby counties. Some 60 per cent of the women, thirty years and over, have had a cytological examination at least once. An estimated 35,000 women are being tested annually. The Society, incidentally, has here a research project in progress that we hope will define a group with a high risk of uterine cancer who will need frequent Pap tests.[3]

Memphis and Shelby County is one of our most well known areas: here, in a program begun in 1952, financed and encouraged by the National Cancer Institute, smears were taken one or more times during five years from 151,000 women (67.6 per cent of the white and 57.3 per cent of the Negro women had tests) and 555 cases of invasive carcinoma and 557 cases of carcinoma *in situ* were detected. "Cytologically detected cases were diagnosed on an average approximately three years earlier in their invasive process than cases diagnosed in the community in the pre-survey period."[4]

Cleveland and Cuyahoga County completed in 1964 what it called the P–A–P—"Prompt Action Protects"—

program in which in one year not quite half of the women of the county had the test; approximately 205,022 studies were done, an increase of 40.2 per cent over the year before.[5]

In San Diego—in a program begun in 1956—about 70 per cent of the adult female population by 1962 had had a Pap test.[6]

In each of these urban areas there has been splendid support from the news media, from television, from radio, from the newspapers. There have also been innumerable meetings, discussions, and person-to-person appeals.

Cancer detection information went out to the people in Memphis by means of signboards and window displays, as well as news stories. Yet just as important as this general media approach was the energy with which Dr. Cyrus Erickson, of the University of Tennessee, and his colleagues visited factories, church meetings, and union meetings to explain the program. In many places, temporary clinics were set up and technicians came to take smears.

There is also a rural county program in Holmes County, Ohio—not typical—where the medical technologist is financed by the society's unit and no charge is made for reading slides.

In fifteen years there have been 44,737 Pap tests made, with 13 carcinomas and 104 carcinomas *in situ* detected. Between 1940 and 1950 there were thirteen deaths from uterine cancer in this county; since 1950 there have been only three. Mrs. Raymond Miller, president of the ACS (American Cancer Society) Unit, gives major credit for success to word-of-mouth discussions and to the enthusiastic backing of physicians. Once the first early cancer was discovered—in a school teacher's wife with three children—the news about the new test spread rapidly and enthusiastically.[7]

In general, our experience with uterine cancer, as with other forms of the disease, is that it is difficult indeed to persuade men and women to act for their own protection. We have not seen any headlong rush toward health checkups. However, there has been progress—slow but continuing—and it has followed careful organization, community support, co-operation by the news media—and most important—widespread personal appeals. People believe people.

In our educational approach the stress is on *hope,* on the peace of mind the Pap test can give. In a special Fact Sheet for speakers at meetings, and for newspapers and other media, the nature of the uterus is explained, and where cancer tends to occur is indicated. The annual incidence of the disease is noted and the Pap test is described as *"simple, painless, and quick."* The process of exfoliation is discussed, and the fact is emphasized that 180,000 women in the United States are alive and cured after having had invasive uterine cancer. The drop in cases of invasive carcinoma when tests are repeated annually is stressed. Concerning the cost of the test, we have explained that it varies from place to place, but is usually about the same *"as a bi-weekly shampoo-set-manicure, or a best-seller, or a dinner in a restaurant."* Early detected cervical cancer can be cured for about $300, while a case that cannot be cured costs the individual and the community approximately $12,000, and a human life. We urge in our general material that the test be part of an *annual checkup* and explain that actual diagnosis is made not by the test alone but is confirmed by a biopsy where indicated.[8]

We have run into problems, of course: one of them had to do with the use of terms. For instance, "Pap smear"— would these words be offensive to women? We checked several copywriters in advertising agencies and asked them to feel the pulse of their female colleagues. There was agreement that women were realistic in such matters and would not be offended by the words "Pap smear." It was a woman who made up the jingle, "Never fear, have a smear, once a year."

However, we learned that our "spots" for radio and television were not being used widely by broadcasters. Everyone approved them officially but no one heard them on the air. My impression is that executives—male executives—were worried about how women would react to certain words. On the advice of our Public Information Committee, we consulted with the National Association of Broadcasters. We agreed not to say "Pap smear," but "Pap test," and that we would refer not to "cancer of the uterus," but to "uterine cancer." We worked out announcements and showed them to the National Association of Broadcasters, which was kind enough to send out endorsements that led to much wider use of the material. These changes seem slight and they did not alter the message but they were important to broadcasters. We have also had the support of the Advertising Council since 1962 for full television and radio coverage—and in several daytime television serials (soap operas) heroines have been faced with the possibility of uterine cancer and many millions have been told of the value of the Pap test through favorite characters.

Concern about such an intimate examination is a real inhibiting factor for some women, particularly older ones. Hence, we enlisted the support of confidence-inspiring organizations of women and of the churches. Our television materials and films have drawn on the considerable histrionic talents of physicians who are authoritative, friendly, and reassuring. During his lifetime, Dr. Papanicolaou's warm personality was a great factor in helping us educate the public.

One theme has been the use of persons who themselves have had cancer detected by cytology, have been treated, and are now well and happy. Brief speeches—testimonials in fact—by women who have been cured and are in good health are very effective.

As with other educators, we have the most difficulty in motivating those with limited education and low income, who have the habit of going to a doctor or a clinic as a last resort. This is a group that has far higher uterine cancer mortality than the middle or upper classes.

In Florida, recently, a relatively successful effort was made to give a pelvic examination and Pap test to 20,000 women far down on the economic scale, who were receiving state aid for dependent children. Florida health officers reported on the psychological blocks they found. I quote, "Several fears entered into the picture; the fear of finding cancer, the fear of sterilization, the boy friends' fears that the sex life of their girl friends would be interfered with, the fear of the girls that an examination of this type would reveal their past activities and others of a similar nature."[9]

Original plans called for reaching these women with a letter but only 20 per cent responded to this impersonal approach. A health educator from the Cancer Control Program of the United States Public Health Service—Ann Rolfe—was assigned to the project and she reports that a survey of the reasons why women did not take the test showed among other things that a large percentage were functionally illiterate and that "feelings of fear and hopelessness about cancer were of an immobilizing nature."

To counteract this, a great effort was made to reach the women with person-to-person invitations to take the test. Social workers and nurses, familiar to the women, conducted meetings for groups of fifteen to twenty. The film "Time and Two Women" was shown and followed by relaxed discussion. Informal leaders of the group were contacted and the Pap test explained. Many of the women were household servants (the American Cancer Society helped reach housewives who urged their domestic help to have the examination). Those women who had the test were urged to tell their friends. About 57.5 per cent of these hard-to-reach women were persuaded to have a pelvic examination and a Pap test.[10] In fourteen of nineteen counties there were small group discussions as a result of which over 70 per cent of the women had the Pap test.

Education for Prevention

Dr. Catherine Hess, now Assistant Commissioner of Health in New York City and for a number of years medical director for the Philadelphia Division of the Society, is well versed in efforts to persuade women to have a cytological examination and in the education of physicians concerning the importance of this program. In talking of her experience, she said recently that the first imperative step was to be sure physicians understood the Pap test and how to give it: "A doctor will not use a technique unless he is comfortable with it." She recommends offering brief training programs for all physicians in a community. Every channel to reach the public must be used: radio, television, newspapers, magazines, leaflet distribution, churches, and other organizations. She hopes to experiment by offering informal block leaders a modest bounty— say 50 cents—for each person persuaded to have a test. In any case, Dr. Hess repeats the warning that winning acceptance for the Pap test is very difficult. It is, she says, "like pulling teeth."

What progress has there been? Since 1937, there has been a 50 per cent drop in the mortality rate in uterine cancer in women in the United States.[2]

In February, 1961, we asked the Gallup Organization to query a representative sample of American women, (837 women were interviewed) about their familiarity and use of a number of tests which are important in cancer detection, including the Pap test. The organization repeated the same study for us in December, 1963 (questioning 835 adult women).

The findings show encouraging progress:[11,12]

In 1961, 30 out of every 100 women reported that they had had the Pap test at least once, 13 having had the test during that year.

In 1963, 48 out of 100 (a substantial increase) said that they had had the test, 22 having had the test during that year.

These figures are probably somewhat inflated. A study for the American College of Pathologists, done by Dr. Daniel Horn, now with the Public Health Service, which will be published this summer in our journal, *Ca*, indicates total figures about 20 per cent lower than the Gallup survey. However, Dr. Horn's study and Gallup's both show substantial annual increases in the numbers having a Pap test, and an almost identical increase from 1960 to 1963 of about 70 per cent.

This table, prepared from a map by Dr. Horn,[13] gives estimates of the percentage of females, age twenty and over, who would be cytologically examined. You will note that the highest rate in the country is in Maryland—33 per cent—and the lowest is in Puerto Rico, 4 per cent which of course, has a high incidence of uterine cancer.

What are the lessons from all this on cancer control through communication? Certainly one fact is clear. The physician is a major influence in health education. This may seem like saying that we are against sin, or in favor of motherhood, but are most physicians continually aware of their responsibility for health education in the prevention of uterine cancer or lung cancer?

Education for Prevention

TABLE 1. Percentage of Total Females (Age Twenty and Over)* Estimated to Be Cytologically Examined in 1963.

State	Percentage	State	Percentage
Alabama	16	Montana	17
Alaska	6	Nebraska	14
Arizona	26	Nevada	13
Arkansas	8	New Hampshire	11
California	19	New Jersey	7
Colorado	24	New Mexico	8
Connecticut	18	New York	11
Delaware	8	North Carolina	18
Florida	18	North Dakota	8
Georgia	29	Ohio	16
Hawaii	30	Oklahoma	13
Idaho	10	Oregon	22
Illinois	11	Pennsylvania	14
Indiana	15	Rhode Island	13
Iowa	12	South Carolina	11
Kansas	12	South Dakota	9
Kentucky	13	Tennessee	15
Louisiana	11	Texas	18
Maine	12	Utah	23
Maryland	20	Vermont	16
Massachusetts	13	Virginia	17
Michigan	15	Washington	26
Minnesota	19	West Virginia	12
Mississippi	9	Wisconsin	15
Missouri	17	Wyoming	16

Total U.S., 1963—15 per cent

* Based on U.S. Population Census, 1960.

SOURCE: Information in this table has been adapted from a map which appeared in *Ca–A Cancer Journal for Clinicians,* 15: 4, 1965, and is used with permission.

In the San Diego program 76 per cent of the women who reported having had the Pap test said that it was recommended by a physician. Among those who did not have the test, 24 per cent reported that their physician did not recommend it.[6] In the last Gallup Organization survey, when we asked women where they had learned about the test, 43 per cent gave as their source a doctor; 28 per cent had read about it, 9 per cent had learned of it from a friend.[12]

Several other interesting points were made from the San Diego program: among women with an annual income of less than $4,000, 42 per cent had had Pap tests; when the income was over $10,000, 88 per cent had had the test. Age was also important. In those over fifty years, 39 per cent had had the test—whereas in those between forty and forty-nine years of age, 75 per cent had had it. Since about half of the uterine cancer deaths occur in women over sixty, this is an important factor.[6] These figures are confirmed by the last Gallup Organization survey.

One other point is worth noting: among white women interviewed by Gallup, 52 per cent had had a Pap test at some time in their life; among non-whites, only 22 per cent. The mortality rate for uterine cancer in white women is 11.6 per 100,000, in non-whites it is more than twice as high—26.2 per 100,000.[12]

There is a home test irrigation kit, developed by Dr. Hugh J. Davis, which is being carefully studied and tested in Maryland, Florida, and Chicago. Here is the possibility of bringing cancer detection into the home, reducing effort, expense, and embarrassment to a minimum, and thus reaching those millions we are not reaching who have modest incomes and who are over sixty—the target groups for the future. Toledo, Cleveland, San Diego, Memphis suggest that a very high percentage of adult women can be persuaded to have tests through more or less normal, conventional educational and medical channels but, even in these cities, there remain thousands of women who have not been reached. An 82 per cent return from kits mailed out to women, aged thirty to forty-five in a specific area is a remarkable achievement. The response from other areas is not yet as high, and is of course being followed with great interest.

Assuming full medical acceptance and guidance, the success of this technique will in all probability depend very much on the communication program accompanying it—in the newspapers, on the radio and television, but particularly on person-to-person explanations that support it. A major effort will still be needed.

This is well understood even in those areas where so much is being done by public health nurses, health educators, American Cancer Society volunteers, etc., to explain the technique and stimulate women to use it. Where this supporting educational program is not conducted, response to the method may be disappointing. Even the most convincing letter is not going to be enough, if past experience is any guide.

One program to which the American Cancer Society will devote much effort in the future is persuading hospitals to offer Pap tests as a routine procedure for all female hospital admissions. In 1963 twenty-five hospitals in New York state gave Pap tests to 9,274 women admitted for a variety of reasons; thirty-eight cancers were found, twelve *in situ.* Extrapolating these figures to annual hospital admissions for adult females, nationwide, the Society estimates that approximately 18,000 cases of *in situ* uterine cancer would be diagnosed if all hospitals adopted the procedure.

Conclusions

The key to effective public education in cancer prevention has always been the support and co-operation of the physician.

There should be a preliminary planning period for obtaining the broad support of the medical profession and the necessary training of technicians, for involving the co-operation of group leaders, and the media of communications for making certain that there are adequate facilities for taking smears, and for reading them free for those to whom the laboratory cost of the test would be a deterrent.

It is important to work out with radio, television, and the newspapers, terminology that is clear to the public and acceptable to both the layman and the physician. Vital, in addition to the commercial media, are the person-to-person networks of communication that exist through churches, women's clubs, business firms, unions, fraternal groups, neighborhoods. Use of such a film as "Time and Two Women," followed by discussion led by a physician, nurse, or social workers is helpful. Diffusion of information is a complex, often slow, process and every channel must be used.

The early detection of uterine cancer by means of the Pap test is unquestionably the most effective public education program in which the American Cancer Society has participated, but one is impressed with how slowly, what social scientists call the "diffusion process" has worked. It has been estimated that in farm communities fifteen years after hybrid seed corn had been on the market, approximately 98 per cent of the farmers had adopted it.[14] It has been thirty-seven years since Dr. Papanicolaou made his first announcement, and twenty-two years since the Papanicolaou-Trout book!

Progress has been made, and all of us—particularly, gynecologists, pathologists, and cytologists—can feel pride in accomplishment, but we must reach the more than 30 million women who have never had a Pap test, and we must go back to those who should have it again. A new health habit has been formed in the United States by many millions of women—this has taken time, energy, personnel, and money.

Reference Notes

1. Cooley, D. G., *Today's Health,* February, 1959.
2. American Cancer Society, Statistical Section.
3. *Am. J. Obst. and Gynec.,* **77**: 973, 1959.
4. Kaiser, R. F., Erickson, C. C., Everett, B. E., Jr., Gilliam, A. C., Graves, L. M., Walton, M., Sprunt, D. H., *J. Nat. Cancer Inst.,* **25**: 863, 1960.
5. Krieger, J. S., "Final Report, Cuyahoga County, Mass Pap Campaign," 1964.

6. Martin, P. L., *San Diego, California Medicine,* **101**: 427, 1964.
7. Report of American Cancer Society, Ohio Division, October, 1963 and April, 1965 (Mrs. Raymond Miller, President, Holmes County Unit and Howard Novak, Public Relations Direction, Ohio Division).
8. American Cancer Society, Department of Public Education and Information. (Facts about uterine cancer and the CONQUER UTERINE CANCER project, an American Cancer Society education program.)
9. Fulghum, J. E., Klein, R. J., *U.S. Dept. of Health, Education: Public Health Reports,* **77**: 165, 1962.
10. Letters from Rolfe, A., U.S. Dept. of Health, Education, and Welfare, November, 1963 and May, 1965.
11. The Gallup Organization, Inc., Princeton, N.J., March, 1961, "The Public's Awareness and Use of Cancer Detection Tests."
12. The Gallup Organization, Inc., Princeton, N.J., January, 1964, "Second Study on the Public's Awareness and Use of Cancer Detection Tests."
13. *Ca—A Cancer Journal for Clinicians,* 15: 4, 1965.
14. Special Report No. 18, Cooperative Extension Service, Iowa State University of Science and Technology (The Diffusion Process, Ames, Iowa, November, 1962).

The Law

INTRODUCTION

The following two papers are related to the problem of divorce only to the extent that one believes that better sex education of the young would, in a preventive way, help to solve this problem, or that more effective marital counseling would, in a therapeutic way, contribute toward its solution. Most sociologists, indeed, do make such assumptions without maintaining that these are the only determinants of the divorce rate.

It would seem, at first glance, that in relating these papers to "Divorce" we have been guilty, at the very least, of a serious oversimplification. In acknowledging the possible truth of this charge, it might be well to define more clearly what we did have in mind. Certainly no facet in the mode of gynecologic and obstetric practice has contributed to the current divorce rate; nor do we innocently believe that by changing his practice in some way the gynecologist can significantly alter that rate.

The frequency at which divorce occurs in any community is dependent upon a great many factors. Among the chief of these is the marriage rate. Ever since World War II, we have had a rising marriage rate, in this country, and it could be argued that the divorce rate has just "managed to keep up."

In the first decade of this century almost 20 per cent of American women never married, whereas today all but 7.8 per cent of our women marry. This remarkable shift is one of the most startling phenomenon of the present century, demanding more thoughtful analysis than it has yet received. As the number of people any of us may personally know who are single has dropped from one in five to one in thirteen, it is possible to be more open in deriding them. The smaller the minority the more total its persecution.

In other words, we have artificially constructed a society in which to be married is "a good thing," and "divorce is a bad thing," although there is not a shred of scientific evidence to support either of these contentions. The pressures on our young people toward marriage are greater than any pressure they may feel to contribute significantly to the progress of our society.

By the time she reaches her late teens every girl feels this overwhelming sense that her life will be judged entirely on the basis of whether or not she acquires a husband, and to be safe, she reasons, the quicker the better. Thus is established the spiral of more marriages and earlier marriages, surely not on the assumption that our country will be better off if we reflect the statistics of India (which has a 2 per cent unmarried rate) rather than the Scandinavian countries (which have a 19 per cent unmarried rate).

We are not proposing here that the discipline of gynecology and obstetrics can, by its professional practice, alter the ascent of this spiral. But we are proposing that this development in our social structure brings to all of us new responsibilities, chief among which is the proper education of the young to accept their sexuality as a reasonable part of their human nature, the proper counseling for the adult who is maritally or sexually maladjusted, and assistance to the victims of unwanted pregnancies, whether it be the adult victim or the neonatal victim.

For such education, for such counseling, for such assistance, gynecology and obstetrics must assume its proper share of responsibility, together with the many other agencies concerned with the total health of our society.

—A.C.B.

DIVORCE:
SEX EDUCATION IN THE
BALTIMORE CITY SCHOOLS

BY ELI FRANK, JR.

Early Treatment of Sex Education

Throughout the long history of the Baltimore City public schools, their instructional programs have never emphasized sex education. During the nineteenth century and well into our present era, our citizens have held it to be the responsibility of the home to impart knowledge and develop attitudes relating to this phase of family living. The schools, however, through courses in hygiene, physiology, and science, have long included topics related to sex education.

As early as 1868 Dr. Harvey L. Byrd of the Medical Department of Washington University was engaged to deliver a series of lectures on hygiene in the grammar schools of the city. According to Dr. Byrd the children were "led by easy gradations from elementary principles of Hygiene, to a clear and useful comprehension of the great laws of their being."[1]

That the schools felt that their efforts were inadequate

101

was emphasized in 1907 when Superintendent James H. Van Sickle recommended that special instruction in physiology and hygiene by a competent woman physician be required in the curriculum of each high school girl.[2] This recommendation was not put into effect by the Board of School Commissioners.

With the development of instruction in the sciences which followed World War I, the physical aspects of human reproduction were included in biology courses. As school health programs developed, school nurses discussed with girls, individually or in groups, menstruation and personal hygiene. It was not unusual for this to be done also by physical education, biology, and home economics teachers. The instruction was not definitely planned and varied according to the individual school. Its success or failure depended in large measure on the efforts of the individual teachers involved.

It can be said that until World War II the home was still considered the major source for educating children and youth in matters relating to sex. It can also be said that about this time the church began to assume a greater interest in the topic.

During World War II, and continuing throughout the postwar years, the schools began to be conscious that the larger number of children coming to them were coming with more needs and more problems, and schools, as never before, attempted to assume the responsibility of this challenge.

During the administration of Dr. William Lemmel as superintendent of Baltimore City Schools (1946–53), significant curricular adjustments, including emphasis on family living, were made. A Committee on Family Life Education functioned for several years and topics relating to family living, including aspects of sex education, were incorporated into the various curriculum areas. Workshops in sex education were organized for teachers and lecture series under the auspices of the Division of Adult Education were planned for parents and community groups. Significant pilot programs were stated in elementary as well as secondary schools.

Although these steps were promising, a look at our total effort reveals that there is little evidence that much has been done on a city-wide basis in the area of sex education beyond the knowledge of the physical aspects of human reproduction. There is no way of knowing just how many pupils have been helped through personal counseling by the members of the professional staff. Any contributions that the staff has made have resulted from an individual staff member's appreciation of pupil needs. There have been no policy statements of the Board of School Commissioners relating to sex education, and no legislation relating to sex education has been enacted either on the city or state level.

Factors Which Have Underscored the Need for Emphasis in Sex Education

There are important reasons for including sex education in the curriculum of the public schools. The increasing incidence of early marriage and parenthood and the problems of illegitimate births, divorce rates, venereal diseases, and juvenile delinquency are important factors that support a comprehensive sex education program for children and youth.

Data received from Health Department sources indicate that the pregnancy rates of white females in Baltimore City in the age bracket fifteen to nineteen years has increased from 4.4 per cent in 1940 to 8.6 per cent in 1960. During the same period the pregnancy rate of nonwhite females has increased from 15.0 per cent to 20.4 per cent. The Baltimore City Health Department also states that during 1963 there were 234 white mothers sixteen years of age and under, and 805 nonwhite mothers in the same age group making a total of 1,039 births. Of the total, 155 were second births and 12 were third births. Competent medical authorities state that:

1. Sexual activity in girls under sixteen is high.
2. Reliable information relating to pregnancy and its cause is frequently lacking.
3. The pregnancies in girls under sixteen are unwanted.
4. Pregnancy is a major factor in girls under sixteen dropping out of school.

School-age children and youth today have acquired much sex information and misinformation from their peers and through mass media. As the child enters adolesence, his natural withdrawal from adults increases his reliance on his peers for sex information. A Purdue Poll of one thousand teenagers revealed that sex information was gained as follows:

32% of the girls and 15% of the boys were informed by parents.

6% learned from courses in school.

7% learned from older people not their parents.

53% of the boys and 42% of the girls found out from friends and people their own age.

15% pieced together information they had received from other sources.

56% of these young people acquired their sex knowledge between sixth and ninth grades and 18% learned about it between grades one and five.

88% of these young people said they would like more information.[3]

In another study conducted in 1960 by Dr. Celia Deschin on 600 teenagers who came to venereal diesase clinics in New York, it was learned that:

64% received all sex information from peers.

21% received all sex information from parents.

15% received all sex information from other adults.[4]

Another recent research study in New York City revealed that 32 per cent of the young people polled did not know that venereal disease can be cured if treated in time and that 60 per cent did not know these diseases were transmitted through sexual intercourse.[5]

Some members of our staff believe that there should be a well-planned program of social hygiene instruction. They also believe that sound sex education is an inseparable part of the total personality and the responsibility for such a program is shared by home, school, church, and community.

All agencies that are concerned with children and youth have an obligation to prepare them for their functions as members of a family now and as potential husbands, wives, and parents later. The school, because it receives all children over a prolonged period, has a deep reponsibility to supplement and contribute to this education and in many cases to offset the unfavorable teaching the child or youth has picked up from various sources.

Planning a Comprehensive Program in Sex Education

The Present Committee. The appointment by the Superintendent of Schools of a Committee of the staff on Family Life Education in March, 1962, reflected a renewed interest and concern on the part of the Baltimore City public schools with this phase of our instructional program. The committee was asked to review critically what the Baltimore public schools were doing in the area of "family life education" and to identify any gaps that might exist. The committee's study revealed that although something is being done toward filling this need, there are gaps in the program.

On the positive side there are several courses designed specifically for this area and many units in Social Studies, English, Science, Home Economics, and other subject matter areas were contributing significantly to the objectives of Family Life Education.

The committee, however, designated sex education as the most controversial and neglected aspect of Family Life Education. It was the feeling of the committee that sex education should be aimed at helping the individual play a valuable role as a contributing citizen in a family situation. As such, sex education must of necessity be concerned not only with the physical development of the individual, but must also be concerned with his emotional, social, moral, and intellectual development.

In August, 1964, when the Family Life Education Committee presented a report, Superintendent George B. Brain charged the committee with planning a sequential program which would extend from kindergarten through twelfth grade. In order to accomplish this task, additional members were appointed to the committee. The committee is now at work trying to complete its task. It plans to present a suggested program to the Board of Directors and Superintendents by the close of school this year. After the program outline has been accepted, the committee will face the additional task of developing curriculum guides and instructional materials for pupils of various age groups. During this phase of the development of the program, it will be necessary to utilize the resources of the Health Department and other community agencies that are in a position to assist.

Considerations in Developing a Comprehensive Program in Sex Education

A school system that realizes the need for sex education must set about to plan a program that insures for its children and youth the necessary education at the proper maturity levels. In order to accomplish this objective, the curriculum must, of necessity, be flexible. Appropriate teaching aids and instructional materials should be available, and teachers must be well prepared to give the instruction. The teachers should be reinforced with reliable information and have easy access to competent authorities in the field. They also need in their teaching the security that comes from the active support of their Board of School Commissioners.

Training in sex education should start when the child is very young, prior to his entrance into school, and should continue in a progressive and developmental manner as he matures into adolescence and maturity. Learning in this area should not stop with formal education, but rather should continue into adulthood.

As the home is the source of the child's first sex education, it is considered desirable that the home should continue to accept as its responsibility additional sex education as the child grows and develops. Love, security, and family interrelations are important conceptions learned in the home. Good home training should include answering factually questions that the young child asks concerning parts of the body or that a youth asks concerning sex matters.

Unfortunately, the ideal home situation does not exist for all, if for any appreciable portion, of the public school population. Since the school serves all children and youth, it faces a problem of what to do with those who do not have the benefit of good home training. The problem is further complicated by all sorts of social and economic changes and pressures which affect the total Student population and underscore the need for schools to do more in sex education for all pupils.

The staff is concerned about the number of unmarried mothers and the continuation of education for these young girls during the stages of their pregnancy. Although some enter evening classes, many discontinue their education until after the births of their babies, or become permanent dropouts. Committee members are exploring the possibilities of organizing special schools similar to the twilight schools that have been organized in other cities. They are also reviewing ways of dealing with the putative fathers when they are known to the schools. This raises the question whether this is an area in which the school staff should prepare itself to operate.

Some educators believe that sex education must not stand out in the curriculum "like a sore thumb." Just as it is a necessary part of family life education, it can be made an integral part of the school curriculum. There are many natural opportunities in science, physical education, home economics, etc., to present the facts and to help pupils develop those skills and attitudes necessary for successful family living. To utilize these opportunities in the most meaningful way is a challenge which faces those charged with the development of a comprehensive program in sex education.

The Role of the School in Sex Education. Despite the increased interest in having the schools do more in family life education, there are aspects of sex education that remain extremely controversial. Our citizens range from those who would have the schools go all out in their efforts in sex education to those who think it unwise for the public schools even to approach its treatment. For example, we have been criticized by individuals who feel that the schools are wasting their time developing a comprehensive program in sex education and who urge the schools to teach specific birth control methods to girls and boys at puberty—at ages twelve or thirteen. On the other hand, there are those who on the basis of personal and religious convictions strongly object to any discussion of contraception.

The committee has now come to the conclusion that the public school system has to take a position in the matter of sex education that represents a realistic forward-looking approach, that reflects the desires of the community as a whole yet avoids the extremes. Until such a program is set forth in detail it seems to me that there are serious doubts as to the efficiency of any such halfway measures.

Again, the committee will probably state that schools cannot assume complete responsibility in sex education. The committee may adopt the traditional proposition that there are some aspects that can best be handled by competent nurses and doctors and others, by understanding ministers, priests, and rabbis.

The success of a sound sex education program depends upon the degree to which home, school, church, and community agencies pool their resources and work co-operatively toward their common objective.

Time must be recognized as an important factor. A sound program cannot be developed over night. When the School Board has time to consider the situation, any sort of awareness of the seriousness of the problem may result in scheduling a consideration by the Board of School Commissioners of the results of the committee's efforts toward achieving as rapidly as possible the goal of a wholesome education in sex for all the children of the Baltimore City public schools.

Reference Notes

1. Forty-second Annual Report of the Board of School Commissioners, 1870, pp. 53, 219 ff.
2. Eightieth Annual Report of the Board of School Commissioners, 1908, pp. 34 f.
3. American Association for Health, Physical Education, and Recreation, New Dimensions for Progress—Report of the Fourth National Conference, NEA, Washington, 1964, p. 51.
4. *Ibid.*, p. 52.
5. *Ibid.*

DIVORCE: MARRIAGE COUNSELING

BY ETHEL M. NASH

Is there a demonstrated need for marriage counseling? What is known of its proven effectiveness? What kind of training should the physician and the nonmedical marriage counselor receive? These are the questions to which I shall seek to offer tentative answers. Tentative because these are questions to which the disciplines of medicine, law, psychology, sociology, and even psychiatry and social work have only recently turned their attention.

The field of marriage counseling has five foci: marital counseling with conflicted couples; premarital counseling with couples about to marry; family life education; research and the training of professional personnel. In every area the demand exceeds the supply. Why? Despite the success of the majority of American marriages, inadequate preparation concerning the meaning of self-hood, of sexuality, of the significance of the responsibilities assumed at marriage, and in techniques of communication is resulting in mounting marital problems. The value systems accepted by youth with regard to sexual behavior are increasingly permissive, so that one can prognose a period of increasing marital infidelity going beyond the Kinsey statistics of 50 per cent of husbands and 25 per cent of wives. Ninety per cent of today's divorces themselves come from divorced, separated, early bereaved, or seriously unhappy homes. The divorce rate for marriages with bride and groom under twenty is 50 per cent within five years, usually after one or two children have been born. Premarital pregnancies are statistically associated with a high divorce rate, and approximately 60 per cent of teenage marriages begin with the bride pregnant. More marriage licenses are issued to girls of eighteen than any other age-group. Marriage bound teenage girls often seduce boys with: "I'll work and put you through school." Somehow no way has been found of making meaningful to them the consequences: the high divorce rate resulting from the educational gap created, and the psychiatric couches filled by women in the forty-plus group who made inadequate educational or emotional preparation for the empty-nest stage.

This situation coincides with the popularization of psychological concepts. In all strata of society far more persons than ever believe that there may be a deeper than obvious source of marital unhappiness, and with the American belief in the specialist they are prepared to invest financially in finding the trouble and its remedy. The result is a spectacular movement into the field of marriage counseling, not only of the outright quacks described in the *Saturday Evening Post* exposé[1] but of often well-intentioned but at best semitrained persons. The yellow pages of big city phone books are well supplied with self-styled "marriage counselors." In an attempt to remedy this, California last year passed a well-meaning but disastrous law which licensed, on payment of a small fee, persons with an M.A. degree in any of the behavioral sciences as marriage counselors. Previously the American Association of Marriage Counselors had admitted to membership only thirty-two persons in California. Within three months that state had a thousand licensed marriage counselors. Fortunately the law is now in process of amendment.

From a practical standpoint the preventive rather than salvage functions of marriage counseling should receive primary attention. We need to educate for marriage. Classes in family life education in grade school, high school, college, and church are a much greater necessity than driver education which puts wheels under the teen-ager's bedroom.

In most states, Maryland being one of six exceptions, the required premarital medical examination provides an opportunity for physicians to counsel those about to take the most important step of a lifetime: marriage. Following up suggestions previously made by Dickinson,[2] Dewees,[3] Easley,[4] and Kavinoky,[5] in 1956 Stone and Levine outlined an extended type of premarital examination[6] which would extend preventive medicine to the new family about to come into existence:

EXTENDED PREMARITAL EXAMINATION
1. Complete Physical Examination
2. Pelvic Examination
3. Dilation of Hymen, if Needed

4. Contraceptive Information, if Desired
5. Counsel Concerning Sexual Adjustment
6. Counsel Concerning Marital Adjustment
7. Couple Seen Separately and Together

An interview survey in 1962 of one-fifth of North Carolina's practicing physicians revealed that 80 per cent never gave this complete type of premarital examination. Physicians repeatedly expressed the opinion that young people know all about sex and contraception and do not want information or counsel from physicians. A preliminary analysis of data collected this year from over 2,000 college students contradicts this. No matter whether white or Negro and regardless of economic status or social class, the great majority want an even more comprehensive premarital examination with specific instruction about sexual techniques, frequency, orgasm, and methods of contraception. Spontaneously they add genetic counseling. Their faith in physicians is shown in the frequent comment: "I know my doctor will tell me all I need to know." Incidentally, they make a clear demarcation between what they want from the physician and from the minister: sexual information from the former; discussion of finances, in-laws, disagreements, personal habits, and religion from the latter. These reasons made clear the demonstrated need for premarital counseling.

Research on the proven effectiveness of marriage counseling is sparse because studies that would yield reliable and objective data are both expensive and difficult. The most extensive investigations have been done by marriage counselors affiliated with the Marriage Council of Philadelphia.[8,9,10] They concluded that both clients and counselors evaluated counseling as having left the marriage much improved in 60 per cent of cases, improved in 20 per cent, unchanged in 10 per cent and worse in 10 per cent of cases. The British study by Wallis and Booker[11] corroborates these estimates. Evelyn Duvall[12] has explored the effectiveness of family life education courses and reports that they were quite effective. However, what is meant by "proven effectiveness?" Clearly one cannot expect to end premarital pregnancy, venereal disease, unhappy marriage, and divorce. Driver education seemed to be regarded as successful in Illinois when the collision rate was reduced from eighty-seven to seventy-five per thousand,[13] since an extra 5 million dollars was requested to extend its scope. Would a similar 14 per cent reduction in premarital pregnancy, venereal disease, or divorce rates per dollar expenditure be an acceptable standard for effectiveness in marriage counseling?

Many medical educators believe that physicians need more training related to the various aspects of marriage counseling but as physicians are already overworked, it would not be wise to suggest that their medical training include marriage counseling if they did not have to treat marital problems. However, two well-based studies[7,14] indicate that 93 per cent of general practitioners, internists, and obstetrician-gynecologists are treating the marital and sexual problems of patients. Only 15 per cent felt that either medical school or residency had adequately prepared them to do this. Ninety to 95 per cent felt that more training is needed to prepare today's physician to "cope with those marital problems which contribute to the current social dilemma and result in psychosomatic and organic diseases."[15]

To advise their patients with the ease and sense of competence that come from knowledge and practice, physicians will need instruction about marital and sexual adjustment and methods of family life education suitable for different age levels. They also need to be knowledgeable about marriage counseling techniques which are based on the concept that it is the relationship which is sick and therefore needs treatment, and that the marriage is itself the heir of childhood relationships. Treatment by nonpsychiatric physicians realistically must be of the kind which is possible within the time limits of their practice.

Thus far no methods have been sufficiently long in use by a large enough number of physicians to be tested for effectiveness. Hence, the following suggestions for educating physicians in aspects of marriage counseling are tentative proposals. They amplify and add to the suggestions previously made by Herndon.[16]

1. The required premedical curriculum should include a course in marriage and the family. Medical students would then have some understanding of the sociological forces impinging on the family and of the psychological and developmental aspects of family interaction. Incidentally, this requirement would increase the prestige of college "Marriage and the Family" courses in the eyes of administrators and when necessary this would serve to upgrade the offered course work.

2. Until such time as this is required the first-year

medical curriculum should include it. Thereby the basis could be provided for physicians from various specialties to indicate how marital and sexual problems become evident and are treated in their types of practice. Incidentally, when a textbook was first used in the first-year course at Bowman Gray School of Medicine an unexpected bonus was that fifteen of the seventeen wives read it and initiated a discussion about the subjects discussed. This interchange as will be seen, could prove most useful.

Material related to this entire area could be integrated into course work throughout all four years of the medical school. For example, in physiology, students should learn about the physiology of coitus. Material related to marital and sexual counseling should be part of the early clinical experiences.

3. There should be provision for the acquirement of clinical skills by supervised practice in taking marital and sexual histories and in marital therapy. In this a form could be helpful.[17] One might also utilize the viewing of premarital and marital counseling on closed-circuit television, or through a one-way vision mirror with interpretation being made during the process.[18]

4. There should be apprenticeship in talking with the *well* spouse in all cases of serious illness. The patient often develops a certain degree of melancholia with regressive behavior in the form of aggression or withdrawal. A medical student can learn in the formative medical years to explain the emotional concomitant of an illness to the healthy partner so that the marital relationship will be in less danger of damage by behavior which otherwise might be regarded as a series of intolerable personal attacks.

5. There should be development of skill in making apparently casual but appropriate comments about sexual attitudes and practices to help couples be more imaginative, ingenious, confident, and understanding in their expressions of sexual affection. This skill usually develops in students as changes of attitude take place through lectures and seminars with faculty, who themselves are at ease in talking about the subject of sex.

6. There should be preparation for work at the community level by exposure to and practice in using family life education materials suitable for different age groups and educational levels.[19]

7. Library facilities could be used to exhibit the many pamphlets and paperbacks suitable for waiting rooms. An up-to-date display could be kept available and students encouraged to suggest additions and deletions.

8. There should be provision of opportunities for medical students and house officers and their fiancees and wives to acquire a better understanding of their own sexual attitudes and practices. Understanding themselves in these relationships will help develop sensitivity to the problems of patients, and also ease in working with them. Suggested methods are making available sexual and marital counseling to students and house officers, their fiancees and wives, and the offering of seminars for house officers and their wives concerning the diagnosis and treatment of the marital and sexual problems of patients.

These suggestions would be useless if added on to a curriculum that was not designed to teach them. Effective training in principles of marriage counseling cannot be simply another appendage in an already crowded medical curriculum. Adequate training can be obtained by relatively minor changes in emphasis and attitudes in existing courses plus certain unifying concepts presented by competent marriage counselors. For example, the way in which the first-year student is taught the anatomy of the reproductive system can influence his attitudes and can be either an asset or a liability in his later contacts with patients about sexual problems. In the clinical years students probably learn more from observing the practices and attitudes of their instructors than they do from lectures. The attitude of the house staff and attending physicians toward the spouse of the patient can be most important. Where obstetricians, for example, include the patient's husband as part of the "birth team" from the time pregnancy is confirmed, students acquire the habit of taking into consideration the importance of the patient's spouse. It is important in all specialties that students be encouraged to discuss all phases of the patient's illness with appropriate members of the family.

In many quarters there is the misconception that marriage counseling requires quite limited competence: less than the practice of medicine, law, or psychology. Actually the task is not only different from but more complex than individual counseling. The view of the American Association of Marriage Counselors is that before qualifying as a marriage counselor a person should be qualified to practice clinically in the profession in which he has received his original graduate training. This means a minimum of an M.D.; a Ph.D. in one of the behavioral sciences; a Master's degree in Social Work; a B.D. and the clinical training required by the newly found Association of Pastoral Counselors plus a year's internship at a recognized marriage counseling training center.[20] Despite the great need for services it seems better to require excellence rather than to provide inferior personnel which in this area of living might so well prove disastrous. The *raison d'être* for everything I have discussed is made clearer in the following diagram which I owe to an obstetrician-gynecologist.[21] (Fig. 1.)

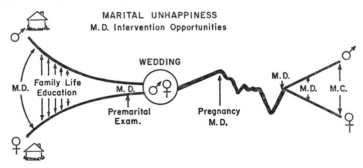

The day of taking the family for granted is outmoded. We need "a concerted effort to help all families in a program of family development which in a democratic society can be seen as a progressive upgrading of families comparable to urban development, economic development and community development."[22] For this the availability of marriage counseling in all its foci is essential.

Reference Notes

1. Davidson, Bill, *Saturday Evening Post*, January 5, 1963, pp. 17–35.
2. Dickinson, R. L., *J.A.M.A.*, 117: 1687, 1941.

3. Dewees, Lovett, "Premarital Physical Examination," *Successful Marriage,* Fishbein and Burgess (eds) (Doubleday and Co., Inc., New York, N.Y., 1955).
4. Easley, Eleanor, *North Carolina Medical Journal,* **15**: 105, 1954.
5. Kavinoky, Nadina, *J.A.M.A.,* **156**: 692, 1954.
6. Stone, Abraham and Levine, Lena, *The Premarital Consultation* (Grune and Stratton, Inc., New York, N.Y., 1956).
7. Herndon, C. Nash and Nash, Ethel M., *J.A.M.A.,* **180**: 395, 1962.
8. Preston, Malcolm G., Mudd, Emily H., Froscher, Hazel B., Peltz, William L., *Marriage and Family Living,* **12**: 104, No. 3, 1950.
9. Mudd, Emily H., *Marriage and Family Living,* **19**: 75, No. 1, 1957.
10. Ballard, R. and Mudd, Emily H., "Some Sources of Difference Between Client and Agency Evaluation of Effectiveness of Counseling," *Social Case Work,* Vol. 19, 1958.
11. Wallis, J. H. and Booker, H. S., *Marriage Counseling: A Description and Analysis of the Remedial Work of the National Marriage Guidance Council* (Routledge and Kegan Paul, London, 1958).
12. Duvall, Evelyn Millis, "How Effective Are Marriage Courses?" Address delivered at the tweny-second Annual Meeting of the American Association of Marriage Counselors, Inc., Philadelphia, Nov. 13, 1964.
13. "Seeks Five Million State Cash for Driver Training," *Chicago Sunday Tribune,* November 8, 1964, Section 1D, P.1. Quoted by Evelyn Duvall in Address delivered at twenty-second Annual Meeting of American Association of Marriage Counselors, Inc. in Philadelphia, Nov. 13, 1964.
14. Ravenscroft, James W. and Kimbrough, Robert A. Report on survey made by the American College of Obstetricians and Gynecologists in *Sex Education is a Professional Responsibility* by J. P. Semmens. Courtesy of Eaton Laboratories.
15. *Ibid.*

16. Herndon, C. Nash, "Foreword" in *Marriage Counseling in Medical Practice*, Nash, Abse and Jessner (eds), (University of North Carolina Press, Chapel Hill, N. C).

17. Nash, Ethel M., Abse, D. W. and Jessner, L., *Marriage Counseling in Medical Practice*, Appendix A, p. 345. (The Marriage Council of Philadelphia and the Merrill Palmer Institute of Chicago have also developed forms for use in a nonmedical setting.)

18. Dr. Martin Goldberg has developed this in co-operation with the Marriage Council of Philadelphia.

19. Semmens, J. P., *Sex Education is a Professional Responsibility*, courtesy of Eaton Laboratories.

20. Dr. David Mace, Executive Director, American Association of Marriage Counselors, 27 Woodcliff Drive, Madison, New Jersey.

21. Courtesy of Dr. Eugene B. Linton, Assistant Professor in Obstetrics and Gynecology, Bowman Gray School of Medicine, Winston-Salem, N.C.

22. Hill, Reuben, "The American Family of the Future," address to the twenty-fifth Annual Meeting of the National Council on Family Relations, Denver, Colorado, 1963.

ABORTION, ARTIFICIAL INSEMINATION, AND STERILIZATION

BY G. C. A. ANDERSON

In considering the legal status of abortions, artificial insemination, and sterilization it becomes obvious how antiquated and unrealistic our legal code has become.

Abortion

There are no reliable statistics on the number of abortions performed in the United States each year. Including both legal and illegal abortions, the highest estimate runs well over one million incidents.[1] The frequency of criminal abortions is unknown[2] and no reliable statistics are available.[3] On the other hand, there are estimates varying from a low 200,000 to a high of 1,200,000 per year,[4] and it has been estimated that in 1962 there were a million illegal abortions, with an incident death rate as high as 8,000 women in that year.[5] In only a small number of cases are there arrests and prosecutions. This is largely due to the fact that the victim refuses to identify

125

the other party to the procedure, making prosecution impossible. The woman is not usually prosecuted since she is not considered a party to the crime but a victim of the crime.

In Maryland, hospitals and doctors are directed by the State Medical Examiners to report all abortions, and are further advised that a failure to make such report is a criminal offense. The advice that the failure to report is itself a crime rests upon highly dubious grounds. In 1964, in Baltimore city, there were 229 reported abortions, resulting in 29 prosecutions and 5 deaths. These figures include only cases terminating disastrously and necessitating immediate hospitalization. The figures are inaccurate since they do not include uneventful abortions, or illegal abortions performed under the guise of misnomer operations, at least one hospital makes no report, and the accuracy of other hospital reports is unknown. To implement the above reports in Baltimore city, there is in the city police department a special abortion squad, and the state's attorney's office has a specialist in abortion to prosecute such cases.

All states have laws prohibiting and defining illegal abortions. In the majority of states, it is illegal to perform an abortion unless to "preserve" or "save" the life of the mother.[1] The words "preserve" and "save" are apparently synonymous; hence in the majority of states, abortions are illegal except to save the mother. The protection afforded by these statutes regards the fetus as a human life from the moment of fertilization,[3] and there are those who regard an abortion as murder.[6]

In Maryland it is illegal to perform an abortion unless a practitioner of medicine "after consulting with one or more physicians, he shall be satisfied that the foetus is dead, or that no other method will secure the safety of the mother."[7]

The penalty for violation of this statute is "not *less* than three years . . . in the penitentiary or by a fine of not less than $500, nor more than $1,000." (In England, the statutory penalty provides up to life imprisonment.) The statute, enacted in 1868, or some ninety-seven years ago, has never been amended. It is archaic in terms of advanced medical knowledge; it prohibits abortions for reasons unknown in 1868, but common knowledge today. Be that as it may, the statute is generally regarded as a more liberal statute than the statutes of other states. The "three-year sentence" has never been invoked; sentences are imposed under another all-inclusive section of the criminal code.

Under this statute a physician cannot legally perform an abortion unless "he shall be satisfied that the foetus is dead or that no other method will secure the safety of the mother." This immediately raises the question: What is meant by the phrase "secure the safety of the mother"? If the words "secure the safety of the mother" are synonymous with, or mean the same as, "preserve" or "save" the mother, then the Maryland statute is limited to the preservation of the life of the mother, as in the majority of the states.

The term "secure the safety of the mother" would seem to be somewhat less restrictive, and broader in meaning, than the phrase "preserve" or "save" the life of the mother, but the question is how far. It has been suggested that in Maryland the doctor's decision is a trifle easier than in other states,[8] but actually the very ambiguity of the statute makes the doctor's dilemma even more difficult. In most states, there is the clear, unambiguous declaration that the abortion can only be performed to save the mother's life; in Maryland, the law may have this same meaning or some other meaning; the doctor makes his best guess, incurring possible criminal sanctions if wrong.

The author who suggests that in Maryland the decision is a trifle easier than in other states, then groups Maryland with Colorado, a so-called liberal state, and cites a Colorado case in which a twenty-seven-year-old mother was raped, became pregnant, and was forced to bear the child because no hospital would agree to perform the abortion.

It is clear that the Maryland statute would not justify an abortion simply because an abortion is desired,[9] or for economic reasons, or if an additional child is not wanted, or would place additional strain upon the mother, or be a hardship to the family. It would not justify an abortion because of the mother's German measles in early pregnancy. It would not justify the termination of a pregnancy caused by rape, or incest, or malformation of the fetus due to drugs, unless nothing else would secure the safety of the mother. In these last instances, the safety of the mother would depend upon the shock and emotional impact suffered by the mother, and whether this shock and impact were such that only an abortion would secure her safety. This rather tenuous valuation is to be made by the physician.

The matter is further complicated by the abortion committees of hospitals. These committees are more timorous than doctors in authorizing abortions and further reduce legal abortions.

"In New York City only about 300 TA's are approved annually, one-third of the figure of twenty years ago. By 1952, Los Angeles County Hospital had shaved its rate to about one-eightieth of what it had been during previous decades."[8]

It may be argued that the statute could be given a so-called liberal construction as in the case in England of *Rex v. Bourne* (1 K.B. 687 [1939]), a test case in which an eminent consultant in gynecology induced an abortion on a fourteen-year-old girl who became pregnant following rape by three soldiers. The issue in the case was the meaning of the phrase—"done in good faith for the purpose only of preserving the life of the mother." The court ruled that this phrase was not limited to saving the mother from violent death, but included cases where continuance of the pregnancy would make her a physical or mental wreck. Thus far there is no reported decision in the United States extending justification for an abortion.[10] If an abortion can only be performed under a liberal interpretation of the law to save a woman from physical or mental wreckage, it is indeed a sad legal state of affairs.

The abortion statutes are driving women from their regular physicians into clandestine operations with midwives, secretive operations with irresponsible doctors, or to self-imposed abortions. This represents a major medical and social problem, the exact scope of which is lost in a haze of dubious estimates and statistics.[5]

Until recently, as evidenced by the attempt to amend the English Act in 1961, "almost no pressure for reform has come from the Medical Profession."[2] The profession has now undergone a change of heart as evidenced by the organization of physicians in New York into the Association for Humane Abortion, Inc., as well as the organization of an association for the study of abortion in California, and other similar groups.

Many of these associations have urged that the provisions of the *American Law Institute, Model Penal Code,* dealing with abortion, be adopted. This Model Penal Code represents a long and careful study by eminent jurists, judges, and lawyers, and in Section 230.3 provides:

> *Justifiable Abortion.* A licensed physician is justified in terminating a pregnancy if he believes there is substantial risk that continuance of the pregnancy would gravely impair the physical or mental health of the mother or that the child would be born with grave physical or mental defect, or that the pregnancy resulted from rape, incest, or other felonious intercourse.

The provisions of this code would probably give the relief desired, and its enactment is only a matter of common sense, decency, and justice.

Artificial Insemination

There is no Maryland statute prohibiting artificial insemination. It is believed that physicians are more and more asked to perform, and are performing, this procedure.[11] There are two procedures,—one is known as the AIH (Artificial Insemination Husband) procedure wherein the semen of the husband is used. The other is known as the AID (Artificial Insemination Donor) procedure in which the semen of some other man is used. The AIH procedure gives rise to no legal problem, but the AID procedure gives rise to the serious legal problem of whether a child born of the AID procedure is a legitimate child or a bastard? If a bastard, he has none of the rights of a legitimate child, such as inheritance, etc. In *Doornbos v. Doornbos* (54 S. 14981, Superior Court Cook County, Illinois [Chancery December 13, 1954]), the court said: "The AID procedure with or without the consent of the husband is contrary to public policy and good morals and constitutes adultery on the part of the mother." But it also held that a child resulting from the AID procedure, with the consent of the husband, was legitimate.[12] In a recent Canadian divorce case, it was held that artificial insemination without the consent of the husband is adultery,[13] and a recent New York case held that while a child born by the AID procedure was illegitimate, nevertheless the husband was responsible for the child's support and maintenance in divorce proceedings.[14]

In artificial insemination procedures, the doctor undoubtedly incurs certain risks. If he performs such an operation without the consent of the wife, he is clearly guilty of assault. If the AID procedure is used without the knowledge of the husband, he may be charged with interfering with the marital relationship. The doctor is under some obligation to assure himself of the physical

131

fitness of the donor and undoubtedly runs a risk of civil action if the child is born deformed or mentally retarded. How far he may protect himself by express contract is uncertain.

Sterilization

There is what is known as "eugenic sterilization" and "therapeutic sterilization." Sterilization for any other reason, such as contraception, falls into a third class, at present without a name.

Eugenic sterilization is performed to prevent the conception of children who are likely to be mentally or physically defective. Therapeutic sterilization is performed to preserve the life or health of the patient.

Eugenic sterilization statutes exist in twenty-eight states, including generally within their terms the mentally deficient, the mentally ill, sex deviates, and habitual criminals. In twenty-six of these twenty-eight states, sterilization is compulsory; seven states do not require hearings, and five states have no provisions for judicial appeal. The few courts which have considered the procedural question require either a hearing or an appeal from a sterilization order. The usual order provides: "According to the laws of heredity, a person is the probable potential parent of socially inadequate offspring likewise afflicted."

The state legislatures and Congress have accepted the idea that the inheritability of characteristics which make a person socially inadequate has been scientifically established. Studies undertaken during the last twenty-five years have thrown doubt upon this conclusion.[15]

With proper procedural safeguards, these statutes have been held constitutional. An attack on the constitutionality of a Virginia statute brought forth Mr. Justice Holmes's famous remark: "Three generations of imbeciles are enough."[16]

There are no statutes prohibiting sterilization for therapeutic purposes since the sterilization is used in the treatment of a disease or injury. Sterilization for other purposes is a crime in Connecticut, Kansas, and Utah. From the standpoint of religion and morals, many people feel that sterilization for convenience is nothing more than nontherapeutic abortion. In the event of sterilization, both husband and wife should agree.

There is at least one case in which sterilization procedures were followed but the wife subsequently conceived a child. Suit was brought for malpractice against the doctor based upon a breach of warranty that the doctor had assured the couple that no child would result following the sterilization. The court did not pass on the breach of warranty issue but held that the birth of the normal child could not give rise to damage.[17]

Reference Notes

1. Stetler, C. J. and Moritz, A. R., *The Doctor and Patient and the Law* (C. V. Mosby Co., St. Louis, Mo., 1962), p. 93.
2. *Proc. Roy. Soc. Med.*, 55: 373, 1962.
3. *Practitioner*, 189: 25, 1962.

G. C. A. Anderson

4. Wall, Leonard E., *Am. J. Obst. and Gynec.*, **79**: 510, 1960.
5. *Washington and Lee Law Review*, XX, 251–52, 1963.
6. New York *Times* Magazine Section, April 25, 1965, p. 60.
7. Code Public General Laws of Maryland, Article 27, Sec. 3, 1957 ed.
8. New York *Times* Magazine Section, April 25, 1965, p. 32.
9. Adams, et al vs. State, 200 Md. 133.
10. Stetler and Moritz, *The Doctor and Patient and the Law,* p. 95.
11. *Ibid.,* p. 102.
12. Strnod vs. Strnod, 190 Misc. 786; 78 N.Y. Supp. 390 (1948).
13. Orford vs. Orford, 49 Ont. L. R. 15; 50 DLR 251 (1921).
14. Gursky vs. Gursky, N.Y. Sup. Ct. (July 26, 1963).
15. Stetler and Moritz, *The Doctor and Patient and the Law,* p. 109.
16. Buck vs. Bell, 274 U.S. 200.
17. Shaheen vs. Knight, 6 LYCV19, 11 Pa. D.C. 2nd, 41 (1957).

The Agencies

INTRODUCTION

Perhaps it was historically inevitable that the devil-may-care, courageous, and individualistic attitude which characterized the formative and expanding years of our country should sooner or later disappear. The great depression of the 30's did much to seal its doom.

The rugged individualist who had loudly pointed to the fact that he had succeeded by himself found in the 30's that it was quite a different matter to fail by himself. Climbing to the financial pinnacle all alone is dramatic, and represents the great American dream; starving all alone is desperate and cold indeed.

We have actually grown up guided by the principle that all men are created neither free nor equal, and we have constructed a society in which any man may fail at some time and some men are doomed to failure at all times.

But as we may have lost our own courage and hardihood, we have—from time to time at least—remembered to extend a hand to those temporarily turned back or to those permanently beaten down. We have done this through our various public agencies, and I entertain no sympathy for the sneering shibboleth scorning "The Welfare State." This is no more than helping your neighbor rebuild his barn after a fire; but our neighbors are now legion and the fires that burn in our society are so diffuse and so complex that we need the skilled help of the agencies to render effective our good intent.

The next step was also perhaps historically inevitable: we have grown to think that these agencies are something apart from us. They are there, we say, to help us if we need help (heaven forbid) and between times they simply encourage sloth and laziness in others. There is no need for us today to underline the real truth of the situation. The agencies for public assistance are not apart from us: they *are* us. They are not to do something for us, they are the means through which we can do something for others. They actively execute what we ourselves should be doing for our brothers, but at no time does their presence relieve us of the responsibility for making sure it is done.—A.C.B.

THE PREGNANT SCHOOL GIRL

BY GHISLAINE GODENNE

This presentation is focused on the psychological impact of pregnancy in the school girl. I will draw mainly on my observations as a psychiatrist involved in the evaluation and treatment of teenagers. However, I will also include experiences I had as an intern in the department of obstetrics of a hospital which served a maternity home and as a pediatrician who several times has been confronted with the problem of pregnancy in an adolescent. Finally I will refer to the literature on the subject.

In order to demonstrate the extent of the problem I could report on the many statistical data which have been published throughout the years, mainly in the obstetric and gynecological journals, but also in social work publications. It is interesting to note, in contrast, the paucity of papers related to this subject in psychiatric and psychological journals. I don't intend to review the statistical data *in extenso* but I would like, nevertheless, briefly to place the problem in proper numerical perspective.

Adams and Gallagher,[1] report that in 1960 there were about 224,300 births out of wedlock in the United States: 91,700 were illegitimate births to teenagers or "a little more than one-fifth of all women who became unmarried mothers in 1960 were girls of school age." The authors report that there was no increase in the rate of illegitimate births to girls between fifteen and nineteen from 1956 to 1960. The annual illegitimacy rate was about fifteen per thousand among teenagers, compared to forty per thousand for women between the ages of twenty and thirty.

Battaglia[2] reports that due to the steady increase of the percentage of the Baltimore population under fifteen years of age: "if the age-specific birth rates were to remain as given in Table I (1960), it can therefore be projected that a 50 per cent increase will occur in the number of reported deliveries in this young age group in the City of Baltimore by 1970. Per year there should then be 180 such deliveries."

Marchetti,[3] reported that among 38,675 patients admitted to the Obstetric Department of the District of Columbia General Hospital between 1954 and 1959, 2,055, or 5.3 per cent, were girls under sixteen. The comparative figures from previous years (from 1945 to 1949, 6 per cent were under sixteen . . . from 1950 to 1965, 5.9 per cent were under sixteen) point out the downward trend in the over-all pregnancy rates in adolescent girls.

Elizabeth Herzog[4] wrote:

> If we look only at the teenagers, their rates have increased less than the rates in other age groups over the past twenty years, and in the last eight years reported

their rates have remained relatively constant. The rates for those fourteen and under have not increased since 1947. The population explosion has exploded since then, and *numbers* in that age group have multiplied; but the *rates* have remained constant.

These observations allow us to appreciate the extent of the problem and to observe that although the number of births in the school-age girl has risen, the percentage has not, so in the defense of today's teenager one might accept the fact that they are not less virtuous than their parents. (It also may show that the education in the use of contraceptives has made some headway.)

Now that I have briefly shown the extent of the problem, let us consider the psychological impact of pregnancy on the school-age girl.

Psychological Impact of the Pregnancy

Let us first follow the girls through the ordeal of their pregnancy and discuss the succession of events which take place and their psychological impacts.

We must consider the girl's sexual life and her first experience with intercourse. This is often a frightening experience to the teen-age female even if the fear is met with denial. The fear of defloration is well known. The teenager who indulges in intercourse, often has no one to turn to to share her fears and to reassure her that she has not been permanently injured.

What leads a girl to her first sexual experience? Many

factors come into play. Some of the girls who have intercourse are often compelled to it by "love." Reiss[5] writes:

> Our culture has stressed the association of sex-with-
> affection to such an extent that it is difficult, at least for
> many females, to violate this association in coitus. Fe-
> males, in addition to associating love with sexual behavior
> more than males, also have more non-sexual motives for
> sexual behavior, such as the desire to please the boy or
> to cement a relationship.

The sexual intercourse is almost an incidental event in
the course of their romance. They do not seek it but
passively accept it in order to keep their lover. If pregnancy
is considered it is dismissed by "it can't happen to me," or
they rejoice in it because it will mean that they will have
someone (a baby) to love. It also can mean to them an
everlasting proof of having been loved by the boy from
whom already, consciously or unconsciously, they feel
rejection.

Some girls run away from home and fall into the hands
of the first man they meet because of their fear of incestuous fantasies. Some are compelled to intercourse as a
vengeful act toward the family. Some are brought to
intercourse by an unconscious wish of their mother to get
vicarious gratification through her daughter's behavior.
Helene Deutsch[6] points out that: "Many modern young
girls have sexual experiences before they are psychologically
ready for them. . . . They are ashamed of their sexual
inhibitions, disown them, and become a prey to anxiety and

depression." I have met girls who are fearful about their lack of femininity. In order to reassure themselves that they are capable of appealing to a boy and of participating in sexual intercourse, they seek it.

We also meet girls who have intercourse in order to get pregnant. In this respect I want to stress the point made by Helene Deutsch that in a neurotic woman's mind there is a split between motherhood and sexuality. The wish for pregnancy can come about by unfortunate identification with a pregnant mother, sister, or friend. Others are even driven to it by an unconscious need for punishment. Some by getting pregnant, test their parents' love. We must also consider the girl who gets pregnant in order to force her parents to allow her to marry.

To approach this subject in more psychodynamic terms, Clothier[7] outlines three determinants for intercourse in the teenager: (1) acting out of fantasy rape, (2) acting out of prostitution fantasies, and (3) acting out of fantasies of parthenogenesis. In the first two instances, the pregnancy is a by-product. In the latter the girl accepts motherhood but denies sexuality.

In the etiology of female sexuality Bloss[8] writes:

> The powerful drive toward immediate discharge of tension is typical of the delinquent, and the age of the instinctual tension-rise is puberty. . . . What puzzles us most in the delinquent is his incapacity of internalization of conflict or rather the ingenious circumvention of symptom formation by experiencing an endopsychic tension as a conflict with the outside world.

141

Bloss differentiates two types of female delinquents (by delinquent he means mainly sexual promiscuity). The girl can either be motivated to promiscuity by clinging

> desperately to a foothold on the oedipal stage or she might regress to a pre-oedipal mother. The girl did not only experience an oedipal defeat . . . but she also has witnessed her mother's dissatisfaction with her husband; both mother and daughter share their disappointment. A strong and highly ambivalent bond continues to exist between them. . . . Young adolescent girls of this type consciously fantasy that if only they could be in their mother's place the father would show his true self, namely, be transfigured by their love into the man of their oedipal wishes . . . the delinquent behavior is motivated by the girl's need for the constant possession of a partner who serves her to surmount in fantasy an oedipal impasse, but more important than this, to take revenge on the mother who had hated, rejected, or ridiculed the father.

In these girls there's no wish for a baby. The girls in the other group who have regressed to a pre-oedipal mother protect themselves against this regression by a "wild display of pseudo-heterosexuality."

> The male only serves her to gratify her insatiable oral needs. Consciously she is almost obsessed by the wish for a baby which in its make-believe childishness, is so reminiscent of a little girl's wish for a doll. . . . The pseudo-heterosexuality of these girls serves as a defense against the regressive pull to the pre-oedipal mother and therefore homosexuality. . . . Acute disappointment in

The Pregnant School Girl

the mother is frequently the decisive precipitating factor in illegitimacy. By proxy the mother-child unit becomes re-established. . . . Such mothers can find satisfaction in motherhood only as long as the infant is dependent on them but turn against the child as soon as independent strivings assert themselves; infantilization of the child is the well-known result.

Regardless of the motives involved the girl may get more than she bargained for and find herself pregnant and doesn't know where to turn next. What is her reaction to this threat of pregnancy?

The girl is frightened. Pregnancy out of wedlock is not socially acceptable. She's afraid of her parents' or guardians' reaction to it and often keeps from them her possible pregnancy. She's afraid of the boy's reaction to it. Will he now reject her and, if he wants to marry her, does she really love him? She also is afraid that he might insist on an abortion which she might feel as a deep mortification, or view as scandalous and liable to impair her health.[6] She has to face the reaction of the school authorities and the fact that she will probably have to leave school as soon as the pregnancy is found out. She's afraid of her friends' reactions, although I've seen girls to whom pregnancy was a status symbol instead of a disgrace.

The girl is in a dilemma as to how, and to whom, to confide. She wants to know whether she is pregnant but again this involves telling someone and when she does get herself to consult an adult she lives in fear that her behavior might get to the attention of those she wants to keep it from at all costs.

Her next step is the confirmation or denial of her pregnancy. In the latter instance, although it doesn't belong to the topic of this paper, I have made interesting observations. Several girls who were very worried about a possible pregnancy related that when they heard they were not pregnant they did not experience the relief they expected. These girls probably had a strong subconscious desire to be pregnant.

It is important to note that the phase of medical diagnosis of pregnancy is often bypassed by many teen-age girls who are only confronted with the pregnancy when they show obvious signs of it. I have even encountered a young girl who came to an accident room because of abdominal pain and to her surprise was hospitalized and delivered. Helene Deutsch believes that one often sees a complete denial of pregnancy if the putative father is an older man. In these cases the man is chosen as a transference father and the pregnancy is denied because of the incestuous aspect of it. "I can't have a child by my father." In the case I mentioned above the fifteen-year-old girl was living with her sister and brother-in-law; the latter fainted when I informed him of her pregnancy.

At this time the child has gone through three ordeals: intercourse, diagnosis of pregnancy, and finally confirmation of pregnancy. She has many more to face. She has now to decide whether she'll go through with her pregnancy or have an abortion. She has to decide whether she's going to keep the child or give it up. She has the delivery and the post partum course to weather, and her post partum future to consider, in which all the guilt about her misbehavior is only too sure to reappear.

When pregnancy is confirmed the same ordeal of informing parents, school, boy, etc., reappears with increased intensity. The child, more than ever, needs support in this new situation but more than ever she's afraid that it is not available to her. Parents' reactions can vary from increased solicitude about their daughter's pregnancy (often because of a sense of guilt) to complete rejection. The child of low social-economic level who has an out-of-wedlock pregnancy is not usually as much of a disgrace to her family and may find herself accepted and allowed to remain within the family circle. The parents of the child of higher social-economic status, although they may accept the pregnancy, will probably make provisions for her to leave home at its first apparent signs and to go through the pregnancy and the delivery away from them. This is often the child's first separation from home and family and its impact, in this especially difficult situation, is often very deeply felt by the teenager.

The question of abortion is certainly a very present one in our society. Girls of higher socioeconomic status are more prone to seek abortion. Is this because they can more easily afford it or can find doctors who will perform an abortion (even to the extent of leaving the country); is it because they are more able to view the reality of the situation and its consequence in their lives, or are there other factors involved? I do not have an answer to these questions, nor do I have an answer to the question on the advisability of abortion. I feel however, that when abortion is medically contemplated it is often with the idea that pregnancy would be harmful to the patient. I can't help wondering if enough attention is paid to the questions: Would abortion be harmful to this patient? And is one answer weighed carefully enough against the other? I had a patient who, several years after an abortion, married and bore a child. She developed phobic symptoms and was then brought to me. She was afraid to leave home for fear that something might happen to her daughter. She was also afraid to stay home with the baby and had to hide all knives, hammers, etc. After several months of treatment the memory of her abortion returned to full consciousness and her phobic symptoms were then explained. She felt that her child had taken the place of the child she had killed and her guilt feelings about the abortion resulted in the hatred of the newborn child. Helene Deutsch reports a similar event.[9] A woman, who in adolescence had an abortion, later married a widower with children. She was an excellent wife and mother to these children until she became pregnant herself and had a baby, when she decompensated.

> The insight we have gained regarding abortion should also teach us to be cautious here: the separation from a child not really experienced in the outside world may constitute for the mother the loss of part of her own ego. . . . It goes without saying that separation from the child will be the harder for the renouncing mother, the more love ties have been created between them. On the other hand, the later guilt reactions are the more effective

in proportion as the mother has felt hateful and aggressive towards the undesired child.[9]

Now let's get back to the mother who carries through with her pregnancy. Bibring[10] writes:

We came to regard pregnancy, like puberty or menopause, as a period of crisis, involving profound endocrine and general somatic as well as psychological changes. Under the impact of the marked physiological and anatomical changes of the first months of pregnancy, the libidinal concentration on the self increases and leads to the integration of, and merging with, this foreign body, turning it into an integral part of herself until the quickening disrupts this narcissistic process and undeniably introduces the baby as the new object within the self. From here on, to the delivery, the second task of adjustment sets in: within a state of growing self-cathexis . . . serving the growth within herself as if it were part of herself, an opposing trend simultaneously develops. This part of herself begins to move on its own, is recognized as the coming baby, begins to be perceived as if it were another object, and thus prepares the woman slowly for the delivery and the anatomic separation. This preparedness equals a readiness to establish a relationship to the future offspring, and this in turn represents the new developmental achievement. [And further she writes] The special task that has to be solved by pregnancy and by becoming a mother lies within the sphere of distribution and shifts between the cathexis of self-representation and of object-representation.

I have quoted this passage to stress the importance of pregnancy in the psychological make-up of a woman. In the girls we are discussing here other factors come into being. What will happen to the baby after the delivery? If they decide on adoption the ordeal of the pregnancy has little gratification. The child they bear will not be their child. One encounters girls who, after having decided to give the child away, seem to try to deny any feeling toward it. They see the child as a foreign body which they want to get rid of as soon as possible. They often increase their activities, start smoking, etc., all in order to induce an early labor and be freed. Some, on the other hand, because they are not going to keep the baby, want to do all they can to give birth to a healthy baby and to "mother it" *in utero*. A girl may change her whole way of living in order to protect the baby she is bearing. She wants him at least to have had a mother who took great care of him *in utero*. The guilt resulting from the adoption plans is partially responsible for this attitude, coupled with the narcissistic gratification of giving birth to a healthy baby. If the child is not going to be given for adoption then comes the gamut of fears as to what life reserves for it and its mother. Helene Deutsch[9] points out:

> The woman's real readiness to adjust herself to a difficult reality in favor of maternal love must not be confused with infantile ignorance of reality and denial of its difficulties. The least mature among unmarried mothers are the very ones who often fight to keep their children. There is a struggle for a possession, not very different from that for a desired toy.

If the mother, or more exactly the grandmother, offers to take care of the baby, the mother-to-be reacts either with gratitude or annoyance. She feels at times that she does not want to share the newborn with her own mother and once more increase her dependence. However, she also feels that she cannot possibly take care of this newborn child alone. If she plans to keep the child without the help of her mother she wonders how she'll be able to work and care for him, wonders if it will make it difficult for her to marry in the future, etc.

The delivery is cause for fear for any mother, especially at the time of her first baby. Marans,[11] writes:

> Many were afraid they wouldn't be able to stand the pains of the delivery. Most were afraid they wouldn't know when they were in labor. Many were afraid they wouldn't get to the hospital in time and they would have the baby on the street or in a taxicab. Some were afraid they would go to the hospital and be sent home because they weren't ready. Many were afraid they would get to the hospital, and it would be the right time, and they would have to stay. Most were afraid of the doctors and what they would do to them. Almost uniformly they dreaded the possibility of spinal anesthesia because "it leaves you paralyzed." They were concerned with the after-effects of the pregnancy on their bodies: "Will my stomach ever get back to its right size?"; "Will the big veins in my legs always be that way now?" "I don't want to breast feed because that leaves your breasts ugly."

With unmarried mothers there is an additional question: "Shall I fulfill my yearning or deny it?" They are "torn by two contradictory tendencies: the wish to be more free and the wish to be a mother bound to her child."[9] Even if the decision about adoption has been made prior to the delivery the mother is afraid if she sees the baby she might want to keep it.

The delivery of teenagers is often beset with complications. To return for a while to ob-gyn figures, Mussio[12] in a study of forty-six patients (thirteen years old) and four patients (twelve years old)—89 per cent Negro and 89 per cent single—reported that 18 per cent had bad labors (over twenty-four hours), 26 per cent had toxemia, and 25 per cent had anemia. Poliakoff[13] reports on 299 primigravida fifteen years old or younger. He reports an incidence of 17.7 per cent of toxemia but that labor and delivery were not influenced by the age of the patient. Aznar[14] similarly reports on 1,137 adolescent patients of sixteen years of age and under. He writes that these patients presented an increase in the incidence of severe toxemia (especially in the girls of fifteen years of age and under), a higher percentage of prolonged labor, and an increase in frequency of premature labor. The prolonged labor according to Aznar may be due to the fear, anxiety, and unhappiness which result in increasing uterine dyskinesia, thus prolonging the labor time.

Battaglia[2] reports a higher rate of perinatal mortality, of toxemia, and of prematurity in the deliveries of mothers under fourteen years of age. The duration of labor is, however, not significantly increased, although the problem of contracted pelvis is more common in this age group. He concludes: "In summary, we feel that the very young primigravidas, as defined by an age of fourteen years or less, constitute an increasing problem of obstetric and pediatric importance, both with respect to their increasing number and to the outcome of their pregnancies."

The weight gain in adolescence is often excessive due to a "jitterbug diet" (term coined by Marchetti) of hot dogs, potato chips, coke, and pie. Marans describes this pathogenesis of adolescent prenatal overeating as follows:

> superimposed on the increased appetite of adolesence were (1) the impetus to appetite common to pregnancy met with no restriction in the girls long accustomed to irregular family eating patterns; (2) confinement to the house alone permitted a constant proximity to an unguarded food supply; (3) lack of adequate gratification from the other teen-age activities added to a low threshold for frustration tolerance served to intensify her need for impulse relief in the available form of eating; (4) eating became a way of relieving all emotional discomforts, unhappiness, guilt, anxiety and fear. Augmented by the inactivity of the last few months, weight gain and worrying were closely related.

Statistical data points to the high incidence of "no" or "insufficient" prenatal care for pregnant adolescents. Bernstein[15] writes that:

> Some studies indicate that the major deterrent is a lack of awareness of the importance of prenatal care. . . . Possibly also an initial indifference toward seeking prenatal care is being reinforced by features of the services offered. Long waits in crowded clinics located a distance from home, perfunctory encounters with changing staff, lack of privacy, and the like. . . . The conduct of the examination can also deter girls, particularly adolescents,

from continuing in care. Despite the sexual laxity which their out-of-wedlock pregnancy implies, many of them possess a large measure of modesty. They can be fearful and highly vulnerable to slights, real or fancied, and frequently need the reassurance which comes with sensitive handling in an atmosphere of privacy.

Although the delivery is more frequently complicated in young unmarried mothers because of the lack of prenatal care, poor diet, etc., Marchetti[16] states that the childbirth is actually safer in primigravida sixteen years old or younger, than at later ages, and he agrees with Harris "that from the purely obstetrical point of view 16 years or less is the optimum age for the birth of the first baby." (This view is not confirmed by Battaglia.[2])

When I worked in the obstetrics department of a hospital in Washington, D.C. I was struck by the difference in the birth experience of unwed mothers and other mothers. The happiness of a mother seeing her child for the first time and sharing that joy with her husband was abundant with one and completely lacking with the other. Most often the baby was not shown to the teen-age unwed mother and she was wheeled back to the maternity floor almost as if she were a sort of criminal. The staff of the hospital was inclined to be less responsive to the needs of these unwed mothers in labor and they shared the punitive attitudes adopted by most of the society. These girls who needed more attention and love, received less.

The question: Should the unwed teen-age mother who plans to give her child for adoption see her child? is much disputed. I would be more inclined to answer in the affirmative in most cases. The eventual separation might be more difficult but at the same time the haunting question of what the baby looked like (was it normal?) would be answered. The pride of having had a normal, healthy baby and having seen the product of the conception may provide the mother with a welcome narcissistic gratification. "Under given circumstances it may be better for the mother to separate from a known and loved child than from an unknown and hated 'something' that only subsequently, after separation, assumes concrete form in her imagination."[9]

Finally, what is the future of the pregnant teenager? If she gives up her child for adoption she may go through life without further psychological problems. However the latent guilt she has about the pregnancy and adoption might come to the surface with full intensity when re-awakened by some external event like the bearing of a legitimate child. If the mother keeps the child the problem of its care remains a constant reminder of her misbehavior. She may be oversolicitous because of a sense of guilt, she may also allow her hatred of this child, who has tied her down to come to the surface. If the mother subsequently marries, the child, however well accepted in the family, will be a constant reminder of the mother's out-of-wedlock pregnancy. The mother is fearful about the child's questions about her birth, fearful that her response to them may engender hate and vengeance, and fearful that the child might run away and repeat the mother's behavior when she learns of her illegitimacy. But this aspect of the problem carries us away from the subject of this presentation.

Reaction to the Environment

Concerning the psychological impact of the pregnant teenager facing her environment, we have touched on the aspect of her pregnancy in relation to her parents. The child may fear telling her parents of her pregnancy but in rare instances takes pleasure in confronting them with it in order to "hurt them." Some children get pregnant in order to test parental love but any such testing is accompanied by great fears of rejection. Many of the teenagers I have seen feel ashamed and very guilty of what they "have done to their parents" and want to keep the event unknown to them.

The parental response briefly stated, may be acceptance or rejection with the intensity of the attitude varying with time. The mother is more likely to become tolerant of the situation sooner than the father. If the parents can view the situation as a family problem that the family as a whole must solve, we occasionally see an eventual improvement in parent-child relationship. However, if the teenager keeps her baby, she might be displaced, in her mother's love and concern, by her own infant. I know of no statistics which indicate the percentage of pregnant teenagers who marry the putative father. Jerslid,[17] however, in a study of sixty girls who married before completing high school, found that fifty-eight were pregnant before marriage. Msgr.

Knott,[18] reported that 50 per cent of the girls who marry in high school are pregnant, and 80 per cent of the boys who marry in high school, marry because the girl is pregnant. He also stressed that 50 per cent of marriages between adolescents have become adulterous within five years and that there are three times as many divorces of teenage marriages than of marriages between adults. Many girls do not want to tell their boy friends about their pregnancy and later refuse to divulge the name of the putative father to adoption agencies. Some are fearful about the boy's reaction to the news of the pregnancy; some, in a spirit of "sacrifice," don't want to interfere with the boy's career by this new responsibility; some suddenly view the boy as an accomplice in crime and reject him; some are no longer interested in the boy at the time of their pregnancy; some want to feel that they have "done it alone;" and finally, a small percentage of teen-age girls do not know who got them pregnant.

The problem of the school is of major importance for the pregnant girl. The girl who is pregnant, or who is already a mother, is often excluded from the provision made for continued education of all children through the twelfth grade. The young mothers, or mothers-to-be, are legally, mentally, and emotionally still children and badly in need of more education. Kelly,[19] writes:

For unmarried mothers—especially those under 16—some continuity of school experience may be not only an opportunity for receiving a much needed education but also the only real hope of staying out of trouble. . . .

155

These girls are too young for jobs, even if they wish to remain out of school. Hence all adult roles are denied to them. They have no peer group available, no means of support, no *raison d'être*. And they are vulnerable to further overtures from boys who themselves run no equivalent risks. . . . Thus when an unmarried mother must forego further education the chances for her social improvement are diminished. . . . All young people need the experience of achievement. According to Vincent,[20] many unmarried mothers . . . have developed a "paralysis of workmanship." . . . Although research indicates that social success has the highest status for the teenage girl, there is reason to believe that social status itself is partially dependent upon reasonable academic success. Those girls who cannot achieve academically may try to achieve socially by attempting to demonstrate their adequacy and success in sexual and reproductive roles. . . . Many unmarried mothers are especially lacking in the skills of communication. . . . Fear is undoubtedly one of the major factors behind the community pressures which result in unmarried mothers being excluded from school, fear that sexual activity will be sanctioned, hence encouraged. But since the boys involved are rarely, if ever, excluded from school, the protection afforded others by putting the luckless girls "out of sight and out of mind" seems somewhat illusory.

Stine, Rider, and Sweeney,[21] report that "in Maryland pregnancy is the most frequent single physical condition causing an adolescent to leave school prior to graduation. More than twice as many adolescent females left school with pregnancy as the stated reason than left school for all other physical or medical reasons." They state that more than 800 school-age pregnancies are encountered in a year in a city of 900,000 inhabitants.

Consideration of Methods to Improve the Situation

In considering the emotional struggle which besets the pregnant school-age girl, we have seen that from all points of view (psychological, social, medical) these pregnancies are the source of many difficulties. How can one prevent them? Once they have occurred, how can one minimize the damage?

Unfortunately there is no direct answer to the question of prevention. So many factors come into consideration that one can hardly program any method of prevention. We should consider better family relationships, improvement in sexual mores, better neighborhoods, less crowded living arrangements, etc. Would the question of better sexual education for teen-age children help? Does more sex education favor illegitimacy? Does the way, or by whom it is given, bring about reduction or increase in extra-marital coitus? Regardless of the answers it does seem advisable to include a clearly spelled out outline of the use of contraceptives in any course in sex education. This would not only inform the teenager of the methods of contraception but should also dispel the fears of so many teenagers concerning some methods.

The role of social agencies working with the putative father is discussed by Pannor.[22] He feels that work with the fathers is important to help them to face the reality of the pregnancy and thus decrease the repetition of their behavior. It also might encourage them to be financially responsible for the girl if she keeps the child. "When the responsibilities associated with fatherhood are discussed with these teenage boys, the overwhelming implication of what they are involved in suddenly seems to dawn on them. . . . Fathers are usually given the opportunity to see their babies. . . . Having seen his baby makes the boy strongly aware of the reality of the problems resulting from his sexual behavior."

The answer to the second question, is somewhat easier but no less complex. One should consider improvement in the family relationships, improvement in the role of the school, improvement in the attendance of teenagers to prenatal clinics, and in the use of social services.

Improvement in the family relationships is of crucial importance but it is too lengthy a topic, in itself, for our consideration.

We have referred earlier to the school's role and its responsibility in the pregnancy and the post partum life of the girl. Kelly[19] states that, in addition to the obligation to help the unmarried mother to continue her education, the school should accept the responsibility for helping the pregnant student receive the medical and social services she needs. He writes that "Even if schools cannot allow pregnant girls in their classrooms, they can—as in some instances they do—provide continued educational opportunities for them" (i.e., the states of Oregon, Washington, and Ohio). There is a special school for unwed mothers in Washington, D.C. Kelly is also concerned by the need for post partum instruction for mothers who have not given the baby up for adoption. (Philadelphia for several years has had a project concerned with this aspect which has turned out to be very successful.) Kelly advocates the use of social welfare resources in the schools and the use of teachers in social agencies. He points out that:

It is almost impossible for special educational needs to get substantial nationwide attention without strong lay or professional leadership—lay leadership often comes from parents of the specific groups of handicapped children needing such services. . . . In the case of unmarried mothers, the parents are either too embarrassed by their daughter's predicament to want to call attention to it, or too far down the social ladder to be able to organize community support. Hence, it falls to the professionals to assume an initiative.

Stine[21] writes:

The problems of the pregnant adolescent require medical, social, psychological, and educational services. . . . Counselors and teachers must provide information, objective opinions, and emotional support for the pregnant student. From school nurses or school physicians, she must learn how to obtain a competent diagnosis when pregnancy is first suspected and monthly prenatal visits thereafter.

And finally let us consider the medical and social help which should be available to all unwed mothers. We have seen that the great percentage of unwed teen-age mothers do not avail themselves of prenatal care. Similarly Herzog[4]

writes that in 1961 only 1 out of 6 unmarried mothers received services from a public, or volunteer, child welfare
agency. She also points out that the girls who receive service from agencies with specialized programs for unmarried
mothers are likely to be in contact with more than one
agency. What are the causes for such lack of prenatal
care—be it medical, social, or psychological?—Bernstein's
review of some of the deterrents of pregnant girls to seeking
medical care should be carefully taken into consideration.
One could add to this the wish of unwed mothers for con-
cealment of their pregnancy, the lack of awareness of the
importance of such care, the lack of referrals of prenatal
clinics to social services, or the poor follow-up of such
referrals, etc. It has also been pointed out that most of the
agencies are geared toward adoption and that the pregnant
girl who decides to keep her child might shy away from
such services.

In order to remedy the lack of prenatal care, one should
stress the importance of such services in sexual education
courses. Although one should work at improving the present services, it should be hoped that if the unwed mothers
were aware of the necessity of getting care, they would not
shy away from it because of inadequacies of greater or
lesser degree. The prenatal clinics should also refer *all*
teen-age unwed mothers to social service agencies or to
social workers attached to the clinics. The social worker
would not only take care of the needs of the unwed mother
during her pregnancy, but help her to understand what
brought her to become pregnant and thus avoid a repetition of future out-of-wedlock pregnancies.

The Pregnant School Girl

To dispel the fear that providing services to the illegitimate mother would be condoning illegitimacy, Herzog[4] reports on the Danish attitude towards illegitimacy:

In Denmark, for example, an unmarried mother is expected to receive help in establishing adequate living quarters, adequate day care for her child and adequate training for herself, sometimes for several years. We are told also that more than 90% of the mothers so helped eventually marry and, presumably establish stable homes. It should be noted that although illegitimacy rates in Denmark are higher than here they are reported to have decreased during recent years. Apparently the kind of help that opens up a vista of stable family life and economic independence does not tend to increase illegitimacy.

I have reviewed some aspects of pregnancy in the school girl. I am aware of the limitation of this presentation, mainly in the fact that I have considered illegitimacy in the teenager viewed as a homogeneous group. I have not attempted to differentiate between races, socioeconomic status, urban or rural population, etc. I hope however that I have shown the extent of the problem and the urgent need to pool all resources available to reduce the rate of illegitimacy in the teenager and to improve the services to teen-age unwed mothers.

Reference Notes
1. Adams, H. M. and Gallagher, U. M., *Children*, X, March-April, 1963, 43–48.
2. Battaglia, F., Frazier, T. and Hellegers, A., *Pediatrics*, Vol. 32, November, 1963, pp. 903–10.

Ghislaine Godenne

3. Marchetti, A. A., "Pregnancy in Adolescent Girls," paper given at the Conference on Adolescent Gynecology, March 16, 1965, Washington, D.C.
4. Herzog, Elizabeth, "The Chronic Revolution," paper prepared for the meeting of the American Orthopsychiatric Association, New York, N.Y., 1965.
5. Reiss, Ira L., *Annals of the American Academy of Political-Social Science,* November, 1961, p. 58.
6. Deutsch, Helene, *Psychology of Woman,* I: *Girlhood* (Grune and Stratton, New York, N.Y., 1944), pp. 91–148.
7. Clothier, Florence, *American Journal of Orthopsychiatry,* XIII, 1943, 531–49.
8. Bloss, Peter, *Psychoanalytic Study of the Child,* XII, 1957, 229–49.
9. Deutsch, Helene, *Psychology of Woman,* II: *Motherhood* (Grune and Stratton, New York, N.Y., 1944), 332–92.
10. Bibring, G. L., Dwyer, T. F., Huntington, D.S. and Valenstein, A. F., *Psychoanalytic Study of the Child,* XVI, 1961, 9–72.
11. Marans, A. E., "The Psychological Impact of Pregnancy on the Adolescent Girl," address presented at the Conference on Adolescent Gynecology, March 16, 1965, Washington, D.C.
12. Mussio, T. J., *American Journal of Obstetrics and Gynecology,* Vol. 84, 1962, pp. 442–44.
13. Poliakoff, S. R., *American Journal of Obstetrics and Gynecology,* Vol. 76, 1958, pp. 746–53.
14. Aznar, R. and Bennett, A. E., *American Journal of Obstetrics and Gynecology,* Vol. 81, 1961, pp. 934–40.
15. Bernstein, Rose, *Children,* X, March-April, 1963, 49–54.
16. Marchetti, A. A. and Menaker, J. S., *American Journal of Obstetrics and Gynecology,* Vol. 59, 1950, pp. 1013–29.
17. Jerslid, A. T., *Psychology of Adolesence* (Macmillan, New York, N.Y., 1957), pp. 283–87.
18. Knott, Monsignor John C., "Moral and Religious Developments in Adolescence," paper given at Mount St. Agnes College, Baltimore, Maryland, June, 1963.
19. Kelly, J. L., *Children,* X, March-April, 1963, 60–64.

20. Vincent, Clark E., *Unmarried Mothers* (Free Press of Glencoe, New York, 1961).
21. Stine, O. C., Rider, M. V. and Sweeney, E., *Journal of Public Health*, Vol. 54, 1964, pp. 1–6.
22. Pannor, R., *Children*, X, March-April, 1963, 65–70.

SOCIAL ASPECTS OF
FAMILY-FOCUSED OBSTETRICS

BY GLORIA BEAN

A doctor is a significant person not only in the life of his patient but also in the lives of members of the patient's family. As persons within a family interact, a changed attitude or feeling on the part of one will affect the responses and thinking of others. I shall consider here some of the social aspects of pregnancy and view the role of the physician in family-focused care.

Some pertinent questions to be answered are: What is the significance of the family as a unit? What social problems are related to pregnancy? What services do communities offer these families? How may physicians help their patients use these services? How may doctors be influential in developing additional ones?

Historically we have been a nation and society concerned with the individual himself, rather than with the individual within the framework of his family or community. Most of us have grown up with this as the prevailing thought. This is a limited perspective, yet in the medical field, due to specialization where we focus on one aspect of a person, we tend to narrow our perception even further.

The family is a unit of society that is just beginning to be recognized by many fields of study in this country. The change is being felt in obstetrics and gynecology, where we are perceiving the significance of the family to the patient's physical health as well as to his psychological and social well-being,

Some of the literature and studies on pregnancy describe it as a normal life crisis, much as adolescence and old age are normal life crises. Observations at one Boston hospital indicated that patients who attend the prenatal clinic seemed more emotionally disturbed than patients from other clinics in the hospital. This was the case even though their histories did not show a proportional degree of disturbance. The profound endocrine, general somatic, and psychological changes all seem to revive unresolved emotional conflicts.[1] Aside from the crisis for the mother-to-be, the husband and children are keenly affected by the changing family situation. Self doubt, immaturity, marital difficulties are likely to become more apparent.

When a first child is conceived a husband and wife anticipate important new roles, that of mother and father, which will involve untried responsibilities and new expectations of oneself and one's spouse. Other relatives and society as a whole also impose their expectations. When there is already a child in the family, he or she is expected to make adjustments and to assume behavior appropriate to the new position of brother or sister.

There are some problems specific to pregnancy where

intervention by the doctor may markedly affect the future well-being of the family. These problems are apparent in all socioeconomic groups, but some may be more prevalent in one or another.

A problem that exists in many families is having more children than are wanted or can be cared for adequately. This includes families with eight or ten children as well as those with two or three. Some parents do not know how to keep from reproducing or are unable to carry out preventive measures. Other parents consciously or unconsciously want children primarily to meet needs of their own—prove femininity or masculinity, compete with a sister-in-law, or carry on the family name. All of these are poor omens for the children.

Doctors are key people in aiding parents to limit the number of children they have. They might ask themselves some of the following questions: Do I have a responsibility to assess each mother's situation and, if my ethics allow for this, ask her whether she wants more children or not? If she does not desire more children and wants to take some measure to prevent pregnancies, do I have an obligation to help this mother obtain the best means of contraception for her and her husband? One study[2] indicates that some women, particularly those who accept their bodies as shameful, or who live from day to day, have difficulty in the proper use of some devices. Doctors might ask further: Do I have a responsibility to follow up the use of contraceptives or refer patients to a clinic or Planned Parenthood office where this can be done?

Another problem related to pregnancy is the breakdown

of family relationships, particularly that of the husband
and wife, which naturally affect the responses of children
during this period. The early childbearing period coincides
with those years of marriage when it is most common for
separation or divorce to occur. This means that help to a
parent at this point may have far-reaching effects. Pregnancy, whether planned or unplanned, can put a strain on
a marriage. Besides those factors mentioned earlier, there
is significance in the man's changing relationship with his
wife as his sexual partner. Some men may act out their
fears of hostilities by withdrawal or aggressiveness, others
by pampering their wives. One reaction I have observed
several times in the past year among clinic patients, is one in
which the husband leaves his wife at the beginning of each
pregnancy and returns in the post partum period. Although
this is an extreme reaction, it highlights the emotional up-
heaval pregnancy can evoke. Since it is quite usual for the
expectant mother to become more self-involved, particularly
in the latter part of pregnancy, the withdrawal of the husband often strains and threatens the marital relationship.

Husbands have reason to feel left out of many aspects of
a pregnancy. Wives see the doctor, the nurse, sometimes
the dietitian and the social worker, but husbands usually
learn everything second-hand and have little opportunity to
express their views or ask their questions. A husband and
wife may benefit from a chance to talk with the obstetrician
during one of the wife's early prenatal appointments.

Women who become pregnant out-of-wedlock represent
a problem of a different nature. The term "out-of-wedlock"
takes into account both the unmarried woman and the mar-

ried one who conceives by a man other than her husband. In both instances the woman may feel quite alone with her problems. From my experience, I would say the married patient, pregnant by someone other than her husband, is apt to feel more tormented; the whole structure of her way of life may seem to be disintegrating and in reality a basic part of it is apt to be.

Whether the person who is pregnant out-of-wedlock is a girl under sixteen or a woman in her thirties, there are certain common problems many of them encounter: lack of self-acceptance, rejection of some of their original goals, and need for financial support. Since the doctor is the one who confirms the pregnancy he is often the first person to deal with the effect of this news on the mother-to-be. His interest in how the patient feels about expecting the baby, his acceptance of her, and his readiness to refer her to community services which can provide assistance are of considerable consequence.

For her psychological well-being, the patient who wishes to conceal her pregnancy may need to ascertain early that she can arrange to do this. In most states there are residences for unwed mothers under the sponsorship of the Salvation Army, The Florence Crittenton Homes, church groups, and other voluntary organizations. Girls or women of any age can live in the late months of their pregnancies in these residences. Many of these homes have programs which include daily activities: educational, vocational, occupational, therapeutic, and individual or group counseling services. Maternity care is sometimes included.

Some persons experience severe anguish in deciding

whether to keep a child conceived out-of-wedlock or to release him for adoption. Receiving help from an agency that has adoption services does not necessarily mean that the baby must be placed for adoption—not at all. One of the goals of an agency in working with an expectant mother is to help her decide whether or not to keep the baby. In some states, final papers granting an agency the right to place a child for adoption may be signed prior to the baby's birth when a mother is sure of her decision. This provides a sense of relief for some women and has the important advantage of allowing early placement for the baby. When a woman is uncertain about the long-range plan for her child, a decision can be made some time after birth. A mother who waits until the end of her pregnancy or until after the baby is born to talk with a social worker about adoption may have difficulty making arrangements for this. It takes time for an agency to plan to receive the baby. Another disadvantage of late referral is that the mother-to-be has not had the benefit of support and counseling during her pregnancy. Obstetricians should be aware that social agencies will help reinforce the importance of medical attention—the social worker will encourage the mother to have regular care so that a normal baby can be born and the mother's health protected.

Some doctors still have reservations about suggesting referral to a social agency even when there are apparent problems and the patient is suffering emotionally. A doctor may question whether he has the right to suggest help, whether this is interfering with the course of the patient's life, how she will accept this, and whether social services will have a positive effect on a situation. To answer whether it is right to suggest services, I ask whether such a suggestion doesn't indicate concern for the patient, particularly when a woman is suffering because some aspects of her social situation are in conflict with other factors in her life? If a patient recoils from the suggestion, the reaction may signify concern about revealing herself, worry about imagined criticism, fear that the social worker will be authoritarian, or a feeling of hopelessness about her situation. There often are gross misconceptions of what social workers do. As an example, one young patient was referred to me because of a complicated home life. Among other problems, she had relatives living in the home—relatives whom she did not have the courage to ask to leave although she did not want them there. When she finally saw me she told me she was afraid I would take over completely once I was in the picture. She feared I would go to her home and personally ask her relatives to move out.

What do social workers attempt to do? They provide an opportunity for a patient to express her feelings and thoughts about her situation in a confidential relationship. She is helped to talk about the alternatives which she sees, others are suggested, and she is led to view these objectively. She is helped to realize that she, not the worker, makes the decisions, but the worker it there to clarify and lend support. Only when a patient seems incapable of making even a temporary decision will the social worker encourage an appropriate course of action. To assist the patient and family members, relatives may be seen separately or at the same time as the patient.

If a patient is willing to talk to a social worker, direct contact by the doctor or his secretary with the social agency may do a lot to overcome the woman's apprehension. Particularly, a doctor's telephone call to the agency in the presence of the patient, one in which he explains the reason for the referral, may ease some of her concern about beginning to talk about herself.

The available social work services vary from community to community. Any metropolitan area will have a Health and Welfare Council, although it sometimes has a somewhat different name. One of the council's responsibilities is to provide information on services available in the area. For instance if a person calls the council, he will learn that X and Y social agencies have adoption services and some of the differences between them, and that Y agency offers marital counseling.

What services are available for families? What important services are lacking?

Most voluntary social agencies or family service agencies offer counseling services to married couples or individuals, often on a fee basis related to the person's ability to pay. Hospitals which have a professional social work staff also provide these services. There occasionally is a waiting list; however, urgent situations may receive priority.

Public agencies, as well as voluntary agencies, provide adoption services. Adoption programs in the past were geared quite strictly to the needs of the baby, that is, obtaining the family history and setting up procedures for the baby's placement. The focus, however, has enlarged to include counseling for the mother-to-be and often short-term help to enable her to cope with her situation and to begin thinking in terms of certain constructive goals. When a woman wishes to conceal her pregnancy an agency will make a referral to a home for unwed mothers. If a woman is not considering adoption she may still be able to receive counseling in many metropolitan areas.

Public assistance funds are available to those eligible for them in local departments of public welfare all over the United States. These funds can supplement other sources of family income to a certain level. The amount of funds in some areas, however, allows only for a subsistence standard of living. It often is difficult for a pregnant woman who depends on public funds to have an adequate diet. In some places, voluntary agencies provide financial assistance wholly or as supplementation to personal income or public assistance.

As indicated earlier, some social services are unavailable in certain areas of the country and others have not developed to correspond with current knowledge and standards. Any attempt to improve social work resources in a basic way should include consideration of the importance of influencing legislation and the planning of program formulation. Doctors, due to their knowledge, experience, and the respect they command, can make an important contribution. Some physicians serve on committees which study and take a position on medicosocial problems. Some are active on boards or are consultants with agencies. A recent example of what can be accomplished is the work of the Committee on Infant Adoption of The American College of Obstetricians and Gynecologists. This group, along with social workers and psychiatrists, studied various aspects of adoption then worked for legislative changes in many states, influenced programs and procedures, and educated medical associates concerning adoption practices.

One of the most crucial points at which to consider social factors is when new programs are being established, programs such as the federally sponsored projects for comprehensive maternity care and newborn care. Here social aspects need to be considered both at the planning stages and in later phases. Otherwise, meeting medical goals will be difficult, since these and the patient's social needs are so closely related.

In summary, the normal life crisis of pregnancy can contribute to or evoke social problems for patients whether conception was planned or unplanned. Family members as well may have problems related to the pregnancy and the changing family situation; therefore a referral for social work services when indicated may prevent further family disorganization and enable the individuals to function more successfully. And equally as important as a doctor's response to his patients' problems are his contributions to the development of medicosocial programs and legislation.

Reference Notes

1. Bibring, Grete, Dwyer, Thomas F., Huntington, Dorothy S., Valenstein, Arthur, *The Psychoanalytic Study of the Child,* XVI, 1961, 10.
2. Rainwater, Lee, *And the Poor Get Children* (Quadrangle Books, Inc., Chicago, Ill., 1960).

The Individual

INTRODUCTION

During the past decade or two we have documented well the status of patienthood. The apprehension at being ill, the loneliness of being hospitalized, the concern over "going to the doctor"—the psychology of these reactions has been the subject of careful study. Also we understand more fully the patient's response to those symbols of power and authority—the long white coat, the stethoscope—and we recognize the therapeutic placebo effect which stems from the doctor's office and his personal interest, or from the hospital milieu of stiffly starched competence.

Since by definition all of our patients are women, they bring to this status of patienthood the attribute of femininity. The feminine role, of course, is an acquired role, learned from a society which defines the term differently than do other societies and for itself differently in one century than in another. This combination of patienthood and the feminine reaction to it is socially created, and it is part of our social responsibility to be aware of it. One of the next authors turns his attention to the impact of this on medicine itself and on the community.

But there is more than a patient in the physician's office;

there is also the doctor. As she is reacting to him—his confidence and his curious impersonality about such personal matters—so he is reacting to her. As she has saved up her troubles to present as a justification for coming to the office, anxious to persuade both herself and him that this trip was really necessary; so he is reacting to having all these troubles poured over the surface of his desk until they run over the edge into his lap, down into his shoes where they squish around as he carries them home with him.

This is, in short, a two-person problem; and while we have documented the reactions to being a patient, we have not always equally studied the reactions of being the healer. Aside from the ego-starch implicit in the mere fact that the patient has chosen to come to us, what are the quirks, the biases which afflict this role? The second paper of this section turns to the other person in this two-person relationship. What attributes should be expected of the gynecologist-obstetrician, faced with the social responsibilities discussed here; and above all, how can a social conscience be created in him—indeed, in all physicians?—A.C.B.

THE PSYCHOLOGIC AND
FAMILY IMPACT OF THE
DISEASES PECULIAR TO WOMEN

BY IRVIN M. CUSHNER

My remarks will concern three "individuals"—if you will allow me a broad definition of the word—the patient, the family, the citizen. While I speak *about* these individuals, I direct my comments to yet another individual—the physician, and broadly speaking, all those who are responsible for his education and training, and all those who work with him in his daily performance of obstetric and gynecologic care. For it is really this later individual to whom this conference is directed, as we attempt to learn of and strengthen our efforts toward a greater social awareness.

Contemporary gynecology and obstetrics has taught for some time that many of the entities which bring patients to our facilities are psychogenic. Indeed, in this hour of self-criticism and self-evaluation, we need not chastise ourselves for not understanding—or teaching—this aspect of our discipline. Textbooks and journals dutifully record the psychosomatic. Many leaders in our specialty, as well as those in other disciplines, are particularly interested in this area, have published widely, and have been instrumental in having this subject included in medical school curriculums and house staff training programs. For these reasons, I choose not to dwell upon the details of these concepts, but merely to outline briefly the psychologic aspects of gynecologic disease.

Generally speaking, psychic difficulties manifest themselves in our specialty in one of three ways: 1. they may be the etiologic agent in a given entity; 2. they may aggravate already existing physiologic processes; or 3. they may be the sequel to disease or its therapy.

Those problems which may be, partly or wholly, *caused by* psychic factors are: sterility, abnormal menstruation (amenorrhea, functional uterine bleeding), sexual disturbances (frigidity, decreased libido, inability to achieve orgasm, dyspareunia), pain (abdominal, pelvic, back), and in pregnancy such problems as neurasthenias (weakness, tiredness, lethargy, agitation), certain GI disturbances (ptyalism, abnormal food cravings, heartburn), habitual abortion, uterine inertia, or excessive need for analgesic drugs in labor.

The problems assumed to represent physiologic phenomena which have been aggravated by emotional factors are: incapacitating dysmenorrhea, premenstrual tension syndrome, menopausal syndrome, hyperemesis gravidarum, and certain vaginal complaints (leukorrhea, pruritis, vaginal hypersensitivity, e.g., inability to use diaphragm).

The occurrence of unfavorable emotional sequelae to obstetric and gynecologic disease or treatment has been noted after the following: tubal sterilization, hysterectomy (with or without bilateral oophorectomy), induced abortion (therapeutic and illegal), fetal loss (including spontaneous abortion), and puerperal depressions and psychoses.

This, the psychologic impact of the gynecologic disease group, represents impact on the patient. Since the overwhelming majority of our patients are married, we are likewise aware of, or should be aware of, the impact of these illnesses on the second "individual" which concerns us, the family unit, of which the patient is such an important part. While I feel that we, in our discipline, have done a reasonably good job in recognizing and teaching the psychologic impact, I fear that the family impact has been somewhat ignored. As students and as house officers, most of us were content to view our patient as a person who exists only in clinics, on wards, in operating and delivery rooms. Indeed, the most extreme form of this shortcoming is to consider the patient only in terms of being "a case to do." Who, among us, during training days, did not become overly involved with the *number* of hysterectomies we would do, the *number* of Cesarean sections, the *number* of deliveries, etc., etc. Indeed, the exhausted obstetric house officer or medical student who sees yet another patient arriving in the delivery suite at 3 A.M. is inclined to see her as another contracting pregnant uterus, rather than as an individual who will now be separated from her family for several days and he is unlikely to realize all that this implies. We have, in general, been left to learn this later, on our own, as we become engaged, after our residencies, in the care of our own private patients. Unfortunately, many of us do not learn this important facet of total care even then.

What is the family impact? What are the ways in which husband and children are affected by gynecologic illnesses? These effects are generally divided into two areas: those associated with separation of the patient from her home by hospitalization, and those associated with illnesses not requiring hospitalization.

The impacts upon the family of separation from the wife-mother are fairly obvious, and indeed, are not limited to gynecology and obstetrics. They are, of course, felt regardless of the reason for hospitalization. However, as Dr. Barnes pointed out in his opening remarks, we need be particularly concerned since our discipline is probably responsible for the largest segment of the hospitalized female patients. The effects include children deprived of their mother, a husband deprived of his mate and sex partner, the household deprived of its home-maker, and financial burdens imposed by depriving the family of its income-producer if the patient is gainfully employed, the cost of medical care, and the cost of a replacement (maid, cook, nurse).

The effects on the family of a gynecologic illness which does not require hospitalization may not be as obvious or as dramatic, but if nothing more, they raise some intriguing questions regarding the possible role they may play in some individual and family problems. For example:

1. What is the effect on the immature child—especially the young female—of regular monthly exposure to her mother's incapacitating dysmenorrhea or to her mother's

emotional outbursts associated with premenstrual tension? How will she, then, respond to menstruation—indeed, to femininity?

2. What are the emotional effects upon the husband of the frustrations of a sterility problem; of his wife's frigidity or dyspareunia or inability to achieve orgasm; of the chronic neurasthenia seen in the pregnant and nonpregnant patient; of the fearful marital and financial problems associated with contraceptive failure and the undesired pregnancy which results; of the loss of a fetus through abortion or perinatal death? How often do we—sitting with our patients in our offices—remember that there is also a husband with the same anxieties, dissappointments, and frustrations as those of his wife?

An interesting comment on this type of family impact, a comment frequently found in sociologic and social work literature, is one found in Bell and Vogel's text, *A Modern Introduction to the Family*. Here one finds a chapter by Parsons and Fox on "Illness, Therapy, and the Modern American Family." Among many aspects of this subject, the authors describe the effects of illness of all possible members of the unit. These are their comments on illnesses in the mother:

"Finally, illness of the mother herself is clearly the most disturbing of all. For in the normal course of events, the mother is the primary agent of supportive strength for the entire family unit. Her illness, therefore, subjects husband and children alike to a condition of under-support, at a time when they are suddenly being asked to meet unexpected demands of major proportions. In the light of this, a mother-wife who is motivationally inclined to cast herself in the sick role may very well constitute the greatest single source of danger that illness can inflict on the family." These comments have even further meaning to us, when we recall the high incidence of psychologic disease in gynecology and obstetrics.

Finally, the third individual of which I speak—the citizen—represents the community in which the patient resides. Here I refer not specifically or exclusively to disease itself, but rather to the volume of psychosomatic illness in our society and the impact of this volume. There is no disagreement that this volume is large. It has been estimated that about 75 per cent, or more, of patients presenting themselves at a gynecologic facility have no organic disease. This is probably too general a statement to be meaningful. The incidence of organic gynecological illness is no doubt higher in clinic populations than in private practice. In addition, a large segment of the "no organic disease" group in private practice represents those patients who have come, because of the passage of time and as a result of our public information crusade only for the annual gynecologic examination and cytology smear for cancer detection. Even with these interpolations, the fact remains that many—if not most—office gynecologic patients have some psychic overlay to their complaint. How are we, as a society, affected by this large volume of emotionally induced or emotionally aggravated illnesses? I present this consideration since it may represent an area of preventive medicine in which all of us might well be involved.

What are some of the effects on society? To begin, I would mention two, which pertain to the population in general—first, the use of drugs, and second, the nature and volume of medical care necessary in the management of these patients. The statistics on drug consumption revealed in the Kefauver report, among others, are astounding by their numbers alone, not to mention the possible resultant problems of addiction, habituation, and, of particular concern to us, teratogenic effects on the fetus. The recent revelation, in our own community, of excessive hospital bed occupancy by patients having diagnostic studies only, with no apparent therapeutic aspect to the hospital admission, suggests a large involvement of hospital space and personnel and expense in the care of functional disease. Specifically, this involvement includes hospital beds which are then not available to the acutely ill patient whose admission must be deferred; it includes an overcrowding of x-ray facilities and an overburdening of laboratory facilities; and, of course, it includes the expenditure of large sums of money by patients and insurance companies, the latter thereby becoming endangered in their fiscal effectiveness. I do not argue that these psychosomatic syndromes do not warrant these studies. Organic disease must be excluded before functional disease can be assumed; this is an essential part of competent medical practice. I am concerned, here, by the volume of patients in the population in whom the stress syndromes exist and who require this degree of medical care. I might further mention the increased significance attached to the anesthetic and surgical risks when surgery is performed for symptoms which are not due to physical disease.

In the gynecologic-obstetric area, we must be aware also of the marital and divorce problems, some of which might be secondary to the entities mentioned today. And the absenteeism in school and industry seen with incapacitating dysmenorrhea is yet another socio-medical problem.

I do not suggest that the answer to these communal problems lies entirely in the realm of gynecology and obstetrics. The anxieties and frustrations thrust upon us by a very complex society and uneasy world do not really fall within the framework of this conference. I would point out, however, one area which could benefit from the efforts of all of the three "individuals" of whom I speak—the patient, the family, the community. I refer to the value of the education of the young female to her feminine role as a possible preventive in some of these psychosomatc gynecologic problems. I ask, then, not only for adequate sex education, but for proper sex orientation. This can be done *ideally* not by the school teacher, not by the clergy, not by the physician—but by the people and in the environment which mean the most to the young, growing, learning child and adolescent—her parents, in her home. We need to teach parents how to teach, what to teach, and why to teach.

In summary, the impact of those illnesses peculiar to women, upon the women themselves, their families, and their communities are far-reaching and penetrating. They require the continued and increasing attention of physicians, nurses, social workers, hospital administrators, curriculum-makers, and residency program directors—in short, all who are directly or indirectly involved and interested in the intelligent and compassionate care of the female patient.

EDUCATING THE
PHYSICIAN FOR HIS ROLE

BY JOHN ROMANO

With the rediscovery, by the medical profession, of the human family and of the human community, attention has been drawn to the clear fact of the social set of the patient and his need for assistance from many health, welfare, and social agencies in the community. I shall discuss the relationship of these matters to the preparation of the obstetrician-gynecologist of the future, preparation which should render him better informed and equipped to respond intelligently and effectively to the needs of his patients. At the outset I should indicate that I support warmly the general notion that medical education, both undergraduate and graduate, should be primarily concerned with that which is basic, essential, and fundamental to its field. It should try always to reduce that which is craft and artisanship and increase that which is profession. Whitehead reminded us that the leap from craft to profession was based principally on dissatisfaction with customary activities and with the trial and error method, to the need of seeing the necessity of organizing and using intelligence in new ways.[1]

John Romano

Does it, then, not seem desirable and necessary to examine the tasks of the obstetrician-gynecologist in those areas of his professional work which relate to that with which we are concerned, namely, the psychosocial aspects? Hopefully, through such examinations, we may be able to learn more definitely the specific tasks, responsibilities, attitudes, knowledge, and skills necessary for his effective performance.

In what follows, I have drawn generously from an earlier statement presented at an occasion not dissimilar to the present.[2]

To the obstetrician-gynecologist come, and occasionally are brought, girls, young, middle-aged, and elderly women. Young girls may be accompanied by their mothers or at times by social caseworkers. Less frequently women will be accompanied by their husbands, fathers, lovers, or neighbors. Occasionally, the physician will take the initiative in inviting other members of the family to come with the patient to see him.

Perhaps more uniquely in obstetrics than in any other branch of clinical medicine, many healthy women come to the obstetrician for educational health purposes and for guidance in their marriages. They come to insure the proper conduct of their pregnancies and, when not pregnant, for periodic and preventive examinations.

Others come or are brought because of the accumulated distress—the pain, shame, guilt, fear experienced by them and by their families as they seek relief from, or solution to, their problems. They seek understanding which may lead to prevention of further difficulty.

They come because of their concern with menstrual problems, for premarital and marital counseling, for advice about contraception and sterility.

They seek decisions about therapeutic abortion or sterilization or relief from concern with vaginal discharge or bleeding, pelvic pain, fear of cancer.

They receive prenatal care and instruction about labor and delivery and are concerned about fetal death and fetal abnormalities and about their capacity to mother their children.

The obstetrician-gynecologist faces problems dealing with the menopause, with emotional depression, and perhaps with more flagrant psychotic behavior; with sexual problems relating to masturbation, frigidity, dyspareunia, perverse practices, fornication, adultery, or with the impotence, sterility, or infidelity of the husband.

And as women and men are social animals, these problems are experienced not alone or in isolation but are intertwined intimately in the fabric of their families and their social groups and with the beliefs, practices, attitudes, and prejudices specific to each.

The role of the obstetrician-gynecologist is in many ways unique in our present structure of health services. He is continuously engaged over a period of time with a normative healthy population in much of his obstetrical practice.

He is often the first professional person, in fact in many urban areas, the first person, to whom women may come for help. They may come to him before they see or talk to anyone else—to spouse, parents, clergy, family doctor, friends, social caseworkers, or psychiatrists. Often they

187

come, even in our enlightened and sophisticated day, because of a heavy burden of shame and guilt and fear which relate to sexuality and to their concerns about motherhood. Patients with cancer are apt to come more promptly if there has been established a positive, confident relationship with their physician, as Henderson has shown in studies of patient populations in Canada and in northeast Scotland.[3]

What changes should take place in undergraduate medical eduation, in the internship, residency, in the post-residency period? Can existing deficiences be corrected, can empiric data be accumulated from which hypotheses can be generated and subjected to systematic study in order to extend our field of knowledge and to prepare better those who *profess* to be engaged in the study and care of womankind?

How broad, how general—or conversely, how narrow, how technical—is the profession to be? I am fully aware that there are many persons other than physicians engaged in health services to our citizens and that their contributions are necessary and significant.

But I also believe the primary loyalty of the clinician, as with all scientists, is to his material. He must grasp it as it permits, pursue it wherever it leads, and develop methods of inquiry appropriate to the material. The obstetrician-gynecologist must learn that which is central and obligatory to him as a clinician, not as a biochemist or physiologist nor as a psychiatrist or social scientist.

He must learn that which is basic, fundamental, essential to his profession, remaining constantly aware of the appropriate application in practical manners of the basic theoretical assumptions and data. He must learn that which is his responsibility, his and only his, and those which are better shared or delegated to others.

In previous papers I drew attention to that which I consider to be basic, essential, and obligatory to all clinicians.[4,5] In my view, most fundamental is learning the specific role of the physician in his relationships with his patients. I believe that learning this role is dependent upon and emerges from the student's basic capacity for human intimacy.

What is meant by the capacity for human intimacy? Is not the capacity for human intimacy a fundamental property of all adults? You may remember Freud's response upon being asked what he thought a normal person should be able to do well: "Lieben und arbeiten" (to love and to work) was his simple yet profound answer. It is generally agreed that this capacity does not appear, fully formed, nor is it ever completely achieved. Individual successes and failures as infants, children, and adolescents—in our interactions with parents, family, friends, teachers—largely determine our basic capacity for interest in and involvement with oneself and with others. When we have acquired this capacity we are capable of interpersonal intimacy. We can avoid becoming isolated or needing to dehumanize our relations with others because of fear of being injured or destroyed.

For the clinician, this capacity for human intimacy is a necessary but not a sufficient condition. It must be adapted to his specific needs. He must learn a new role, constituting the means to an end, not an end in itself. It is a role which requires interest in and capacity for involvement with self and with others. Also necessary is conscious awareness of the implicit mutual expectations and emotional attitudes of the clinician and his patient. The role must be learned through example and through precept. The clinician must acquire compassionate objectivity in order to observe clearly and reliably, and record accurately so that the inferences from his observations may be valid and his decisions wise.

Can the events of this human interaction affect significantly the perceptual field of the clinician? Can it restrict or stretch his mechanism for gathering information? The patient, she who suffers, whether it be from bleeding, discharge, pain, comes or occasionally is taken to the physician, from whom is expected relief of distress, if not understanding leading to prevention. Can the fact of this interaction with the implicit mutual expectations and emotional attitudes affect not only the clinician's information gathering process, but the manner in which he draws inferences and makes decisions from such information? Is this knowledge to be left to chance? Is the clinician of tomorrow to depend solely, as has his predecessor, on his personal idiosyncratic sampling of human experience?

I have the impression that the relationship between the obstetrician-gynecologist and his patient may have certain qualitative differences as compared with the relations between other physicians and their patients. While I am aware that obstetrics-gynecology is not the only clinical discipline that carries with it both medical and surgical responsibilities, this fact may have special significance. The obstetrician-gynecologist is required to learn a broad array of attitudes and adaptive sets as he deals with his patients. At one extreme he must retain the objectivity so necessary for surgical performance. At the other he must be sensitive to and perceptive of the highly emotional situations of his patients in dealing with problems relating to sexual and social conduct. When a physician has the need for only one set of adaptive devices, it is easier to learn them, and one avoids the constant changes necessary when one assumes different postures and responsibilities.

Another characteristic relates to the problems the obstetrician-gynecologist faces in dealing with his anxieties and shames and guilts in fulfilling his specific responsibilities. He is confronted more directly than are most physicians with the realistic need to look at and touch the genitals of his patients, to learn of their sexual practices, and to advise them in these matters. It is not easy to avoid the extremes of denial or sequestration or, at the other end, of exaggerated overidentification. The problem, of course, is universal to all physicians. I draw attention only to its special qualities in this field.

In my view, one of the most significant contributions the obstetrician-gynecologist can make in his daily practice is to intervene appropriately, skillfully, and intelligently in crisis situations. A crisis situation has been defined as a state of disequilibrium, a state of imbalance.[6] It may become manifest in behavior which is predominantly biological, psychological, or social, and oftentimes with combinations of these. It appears as a phase of unrest in a person who previously has maintained a relatively stable state. It is not static. The person involved is not yet necessarily sick or diseased. The situation precedes or is the precursor to psychopathology. Resolution of the crisis may lead to adaptive, integrative behavior, that is, to mastery of the issue being confronted or else to maladaptive disintegrative behavior, to sickness or disease.

The obstetrician-gynecologist is in a unique position to help his patients at points of crisis. I believe that crisis situations are more common and have special importance in obstetrics and gynecology because of the pervasive conscious or unconscious concern with sexual functions and with the functions of mothering. Consider these three instances, for example:

1. The teen-age girl concerned with delayed menarche, irregular periods, unexplained bleeding, discharge—her mind deluged with fear, confusion, ignorance about sexual matters—both factual and fancied.

2. The menopausal woman concerned with cancer fear, with impending nervousness or craziness, but most often with a basic dread of loss of femininity and sexual attractiveness, of a change in body image.

3. Women confronted with the stark fact of the unsuccessful termination of pregnancy—whether due to abortion, prematurity, fetal death—with the sadness, perplexity, anger, and shame of "Am I found wanting as a woman—what is wrong with me?"

I believe the number of such experiences is legion. I believe one can learn to deal with these directly, intelligently, and skillfully through the understanding, intervention, and support of the obstetrician and gynecologist. If there is delay or mismanagement, there may be the danger of the development of maladaptive neurotic and psychosomatic symptom formation, at times becoming thickly encrusted, difficult to reach—often producing chronic disability and invalidism.

Psychiatrists are in urgent need of additional information. The obstetrician-gynecologist has a uniquely rich opportunity to inform them and to add immeasurably to the number and accuracy of primary data. There are many areas of human behavior about which psychiatrists have, at best, limited information, or information obtained quite often retrospectively. They include:

1. Empiric psychobiologic data of menstrual functions including psychosocial attitudes about menarche, dysfunction, fertility, sterilization, menopause.

2. Empiric psychobiologic data of the sexual response of the human female.[7]

3. Changing attitudes toward and practices of sexual behavior, marriage, parenthood, and number of children.

4. Experiences with genetic counseling.

5. Normative emotional experience of women intra- and post partum with particular attention to the post partum psychosis.

6. Empiric data of maternal reactions to fetal death or abnormality in the nature of grief and grieving, the adaptive and maladaptive responses of parents and family.

7. Data concerning contraceptive practices, artificial insemination, of indications for therapeutic abortion and sterilization, including the after effects of these in the lives

of women and their husbands, such as remorse, anger, guilt, shame, or relief.

8. Significance of pelvic pain, of multiple elective operative intervention in certain patients as modes of dealing with emotional problems, of postoperative agitated depressive reactions to pelvic surgery.

9. Empiric data of mothers of living children who had unsuccessfully attempted to abort, who manifest shame and guilt and who may contribute to the vulnerable child syndrome.

10. Normative data of psychologic and social impact of black, grey, and white adoption markets, the psychology of separation, loss, and giving up; the psychology of the decisions made by the obstetrician in adoption and of his relations with the natural mother, prospective parents, social caseworkers, and social agencies.

Much of what is subsumed in these could provide data for intelligent and enlightened social action in matters relating to contraception, fertility, abortion. Much, too, would be highly relevant to the promotion of preventive medicine.

Studies of these problems and of others would add materially to a basic core of normative data, that is, to a set of baselines from which we could make more intelligent clinical judgments. For example, is there such an entity as the "post partum blues?" Does this exist, and, if so, what are its characteristic properties, its incidence and prevalence, its course? What are its variations, and is it modifiable? What is its relation to the much-dreaded post partum psychosis?

The immediate practical value of this information, which many obstetrician-gynecologists must have acquired, would be of tremendous help to the psychiatrist when he is asked to make his clinical judgment.

I refer briefly to a study about to be completed by Frederick Melges, a psychiatric house officer at Strong Memorial Hospital. He studied 100 women patients whose psychiatric illness began in the period one month pre partum to three months post partum. He was able to examine 74 of the 100 women personally. Let me list some of his most significant findings:

1. Thirty-five patients had been given a definite psychiatric diagnosis in the past.

2. There was a prominent repetitive pattern of severe post partum blues or psychosis.

3. Fifty-seven per cent of the patients had a positive family history of mental illness, and over 50 per cent reported post partum psychic reactions in their women relatives.

4. Sixty-four per cent had the onset of psychic symptoms within the first ten days post partum. The median onset was four days post partum.

5. The most prominent clinical symptomatology was a confusional state, unlike classical delirium, but with evidences of identity diffusion.

6. Conflict over mothering constituted a major precipitating stress in 68 per cent of the patients. There appeared to be a repudiation of the mothering role because of an ambivalent identification with a controlling-rejecting mother; 58 per cent of the patients' mothers were described

as both controlling and rejecting, 80 per cent as rejecting, 73 per cent as controlling.

7. A great number of the patients' mothers had received psychiatric care (over 30 per cent); 13 per cent were psychotic at one time.

It appeared that the nature of the clinical symptomatology with guilt, depression, and perplexity, had some relationship to the patient's identification with her controlling-rejecting mother. At a critical time, when the patient is to assume a mothering role, the nature of this earlier identification is reactivated and appears to induce the patient to reject her own infant, similar to her own mother's rejecting attitude toward her. The confusion, guilt, depression, and perplexity which ensues appears to be enhanced if there is no positive rallying figure in the home to help the new mother to correct and to modify her earlier set patterns.

The preventive, as well as diagnostic significance of Melges' study points to the need for obstetrician-gynecologists to learn more from their patients of previous mental illnesses in the patients' mothers, as well as of their patients, of the nature of the past and present relationship between the patient and her mother, and the nature of the home setting to which the patient is to return with her baby. In our view, such information could lead to constructive advice during the pregnancy, during the conduct of the labor, and to certain supportive provisions in the home when the patient returns to it with her baby.[8]

It is my view that the obstetrician-gynecologist is in a unique position himself to make observations, accumulate data, and transmit them to others. I do not mean that he should become a social scientist or psychiatrist, no more than I think he should become primarily an anatomist or biochemist. I do believe he must learn the methods and techniques, acquire the knowledge and skills which are necessary to his task. He must learn, then, from psychology and the social sciences, just as he learns from morphology, chemistry, and physiology that which is central and basic to his work. Each is a science basic to his role as an obstetrician-gynecologist. How can the clinician survive if he insists on systematic knowledge in one aspect of his work but is content with intuitive-artistic, most frequently nontransmissible knowledge in another?

There appears to be little question that in the immediate future there will occur a much more intimate intellectual relationship between genetics, embryology, and the sciences referable to growth and development in the undergraduate medical curriculum, and that obstetrics and gynecology will and should take part vigorously in this development.[9,10] The increased interest and intensity of researches on the part of obstetricians-gynecologists in the morphology, chemistry, and physiology of the placenta and the fetus attest to this. It seems likely that this development will be reflected in changes in the traditional undergraduate and graduate teaching in obstetrics and gynecology. Is it possible that because of comparable changes in undergraduate medical teaching stemming from psychology and the social sciences through the media of psychiatry, preventive medicine, and obstetrics-gynecology itself, that these, too, may be reflected eventually in changes in traditional obstetric-gynecologic teaching? Similarly at the graduate level, it seems likely that there will be a more intimate development between psychology, psychiatry, and the social sciences and the field of obstetrics and gynecology.

If these predictions prove to be correct, models and exemplars may emerge—teachers, investigators, and clinical practitioners in the field of obstetrics and gynecology who are different from many of the models currently recognized as being primarily concerned with technical and manipulative matters.

May it happen that from these two sources, one from physical, chemical biology, the other from psychosocial biology, there may develop a broadening of the fields now called obstetrics and gynecology. Perhaps there will evolve a broader clinical science, most appropriately called "gynecology" not only in its current meaning, "that department of medical science which treats of the functions and diseases peculiar to women," but in a larger sense to its fuller meaning, namely, toward a science of womankind.

The moment is propitious. In a sense it is a time of crisis. Justice Douglas reminds us that when the Chinese write the word "crisis," they do so in two characters, one of which means "danger" and the other "opportunity." If we have learned our lesson properly, we know that we must act intelligently and appropriately at a moment of crisis. It appears to me that at one extreme the profession may choose to become more restrictive, in a sense more technical and manipulative. At the other, it may point toward the larger dimension of a science of womankind. What will happen will depend in great part on which the leaders in this profession decide. Much will depend, too, on the image presented to young students and to those attracted to join the specialty in the exciting years to come.

Reference Notes

1. Whitehead, A. N., *Adventures of Ideas* (Great Britain: Pelican Books, 1948).
2. Romano, J., *Bulletin of the Sloane Hospital for Women,* X: 267–74, Winter, 1964.
3. Henderson, J. G., Wittkower, E. D., Lougheed, M. N., *J. Psychosomatic Res.,* 3: 27–41, 1958.
   Henderson, J. G., "Denial and Repression as Factors in the Delay of Patients with Cancer Presenting to the Physician," to be published with proceedings of the Conference on Psychophysiological Aspects of Cancer, The New York Academy of Sciences, April, 1965.
4. Romano, J., *Journal of Medical Education,* 38: 584–90, 1963.
5. Romano, J., *J.A.M.A.,* 190: 282–84, 1964.
6. Marmor, J., "Role of Psychoanalysis in Programs of Prevention in Mental Health." Summary of unpublished Proceedings, National Institute Mental Health, March, 1961.
7. Masters, William H., *Western Journal of Surgery, Obstetrics and Gynecology,* 70: 248–57, 1962.
8. Melges, F., "Studies of Patients with Post-partum Psychosis" (unfinished work).
9. Kimbrough, R. A., Miller, Norman F., Barnes, Allan C., Parks, John, Taylor, E. Stewart, and McKelvey, I. L., *American Journal of Obstetrics and Gynecology,* 84: 1160–76, 1962.
10. Taylor, H. C., Jr., *The Recruitment of Talent for a Medical Specialty* (C. V. Mosby Co., St. Louis, Mo., 1961).

COMMENTARY

By Dr. Barnes

The final paper has turned to our need to educate the physician. But from the preceding ones discussing our social needs, a pattern begins to emerge.

We see a globe that needs to be motivated to restrict its growth, but we are surrounded by nations that must motivate themselves. This is not simply a verbal dilemma; this is the acknowledged way of the world. In the face of the population problem outlined earlier, achieving such motivation is imperative. It will require the leadership of governments, but also the support of the people.

Whether as physician or as citizen, one should not await "the perfect method" of conception control before raising one's voice. There is no guarantee that any better methods than those outlined here will ever be discovered. Some degree of failure may well attend all contraceptive techniques, which fact should be no cause for alarm: we are seeking not the complete "cure" of reproduction, but its sensible control.

In our more immediate neighborhoods, we need a school system which will more effectively aid in sex education, and we have had indicated the need for education in contraception. We likewise need a school system, or some other social provision, which will continue to educate the pregnant school girl. Providing that girl second-class prenatal care and denying to her continuing educational opportunities—in the face of the unhappy results whose evidence is here presented—are not social gestures calculated to improve either the maternal or the neonatal citizen.

The pattern seems to call for some legal revision, since we have laws with respect to abortion, sterilization, and artificial insemination which are antiquated and unrealistic. The existence of these is often acknowledged by the gynecologist-obstetrician more by the breach than by the observance, which nevertheless leaves him carrying singly the burden of legal risk, and reduces our efforts at either social control or biologic improvement to the relatively clandestine and occasional, where they should be open and massively mounted.

Directly or indirectly many of these papers have brought us to the question of the civil rights of the fetus. Have you and I the right to condemn him to be born to dirt and squalor, into a family which does not want him, cannot afford him, and will totally neglect him? Have we the right to force the anomalous to be born, even when his defect can be diagnosed months before term? Must we await the miraculous appearance of a neonatal Thomas Jefferson, or is it a part of *our* social responsibility to compose a new Bill of Rights?

EPILOGUE

This conference does not need, in the customary sense of the word, a summarization. On the other hand, such diverse individual topics could well be brought back to a focal point, and our initial premise re-examined.

We have, from start to finish, been discussing people— people banded together in communities, huddled together on a shrinking globe, housed together in a family, people lonely in a hospital bed, but always individual people.

Medicine is one aspect of individual man's eternal effort to understand and to conquer his environment. Indeed, all science and all scientific research, as well as the law itself, are part of this effort. It is apparent to everyone, however, that this effort may have backfired, may have, in fact, led us the wrong direction. Because we have with our contemporary science and our legalism not only conquered much of our environment, we have also created an environment. And looking at the tensions, noises, fumes, bombs, and threats of extinction implicit in this new environment it becomes equally apparent that we have created a world which might in truth be incompatible with our biologic existence in the happiest sense. There is no guarantee that man can stand indefinite deprivation, mechanization, crowding, and the imminent threat of dissolution; indeed there is some good evidence that the biologic system has a top limit, a peak load of what it can withstand without crumbling into chronic adrenal insufficiency from an eternal stress reaction.

We live in a society which is shooting at us, and the bullets strike us and our patients in almost a random fashion. We call the bullet wounds ulcers, menstrual irregularity, pelvic pain, frigidity, psychoneurosis—and we bind up each wound as though it were an isolated medical event rather than recognizing it as always part of a larger struggle.

But it is, indeed, a larger struggle—a struggle implicit in the weapon which has turned in our hands; the Frankenstein which was meant to conquer the environment has created an environment, and we have nothing left with which to defend ourselves in this new milieu.

This is the responsibility of gynecology and obstetrics, and of medical education, and of medicine; but it is also the responsibility of all of us. We have not solved that problem in this conference, but our initial quest was not the blue-print of an immediate solution. We set out to recognize the problem, delineate it, explore some of its facets, and this, I think, we have done.

A society more compatible with both our biologic limitations and our biologic advantages may some day emerge, but we did not necessarily set out to create it today. This discipline can prescribe medications for the pelvic pain, support the insecurity and the crippled ego which lies back of that pain. But today we were pausing to recognize that we live in a society in which these pains and related symptoms are endemic, and that the injured ego is no more the cause of the patient's distress than are bullets the cause of war.

We are, in a sense, a society of the walking wounded, collectively overcrowded and individually hurt, and the correction of this situation is the urgent task to which we should commit our thoughtful energies. The time to start was yesterday—A.C.B.

INDEX

206

Index

Index

Helvetius, 61
Henderson, 188
Herndon, 118
Herzog, Elizabeth, 138, 159, 161
Hess, Dr. Catherine, 89
Higher Horizons Project: intellectual resuscitation, 69
Hobbes, Thomas, 58, 59
Holmes County study: cancer detection, 84
Holmes, Mr. Justice, 133
Horn, Dr. Daniel, 90
Hubel, 63
Human betterment, 70
Human reproduction courses, 102

Illegitimacy rate, 138
Incon, 21 ff.
India: contraception, 9; population increase, 28; family size, 30, 33, 35; unmarried rate, 98
Indianapolis study: contraception, 35, 36
Infanticide, 31
Intrauterine contraceptive devices, 9, 16 ff., 20, 32, 37
I. Q., 60, 66, 68

Jamaica: motivations for contraception, 35
Japan: population growth, 6, 31
Jerslid, 154
Jitterbug diet, 151
Johns Hopkins Hospital, xiv, 16, 19
Justifiable abortion, 130

Kansas, sterilization, 133
Kavinoky, 115
Kefauver report on drug consumption, 183
Kelly, 155, 158
Knott, 155
Korea: intrauterine contraceptive devices in, 32
Kwashinokor (protein deficiency disease), 12

Latin American population growth, 6, 7, 10, 12
Law, 97; English abortion, 126; Maryland abortion, 127
Law of Nature, 59
Lemmel, Dr. William, 102

Manhattan Project: population crisis, 13
Marans, 149, 151
Marchetti, 138, 151, 152
Marital counseling, 97, 113; North Carolina survey, 116
Marriage Council of Philadelphia, 116
Marriage Counselors, American Association of, 115, 121
Maryland abortion law, 90, 115, 126
Maryland State Medical Examiners: re reporting abortions, 126
Maternal mortality, 43, 44; uterine cancer, 81, 82
Meier, 34
Melges, Frederick: psychiatric study of pre and post partum women, 195, 196
Miller, Mrs. Raymond, 84
Model Penal Code: re justifiable abortion, 130
Mortality, perinatal, 34
Mussio, 150

Nash, Ethel M., 113
National Association of Broadcasters: re Pap tests, 86
National Cancer Institute, 81, 83
Nature, State of, 59
Neoplasia: control of, 75; education for prevention of, 79
Newton, 60
Nissen, 63
North Carolina survey on marital counseling, 116

Obstetrician-gynecologist and psychiatrist: interrelationship, 193

208

Index

209

Index

THE SOCIAL RESPONSIBILITY OF GYNECOLOGY AND OBSTETRICS

EDITED AND WITH INTRODUCTIONS BY ALLAN C. BARNES

designer: Edward King
typesetter: Monotype Composition Company
typefaces: Fairfield, Perpetua
printer: John D. Lucas Printing Company
paper: Warren Old Style Antique Laid Finish
binder: Moore and Company